CHEMICAL ENGINEERING METHODS AND TECHNOLOGY

XENOBIOTICS: NEW RESEARCH

CHEMICAL ENGINEERING METHODS AND TECHNOLOGY

Additional books in this series can be found on Nova's website under the Series tab.

Additional e-books in this series can be found on Nova's website under the e-book tab.

BIOCHEMISTRY RESEARCH TRENDS

Additional books in this series can be found on Nova's website under the Series tab.

Additional e-books in this series can be found on Nova's website under the e-book tab.

CHEMICAL ENGINEERING METHODS AND TECHNOLOGY

XENOBIOTICS: NEW RESEARCH

SAUL F. CASTANEDA

AND

MAURO L. EMERSON

EDITORS

Nova Science Publishers, Inc.

New York

LIBRARY OF CONGRESS CATALOGING-IN-PUBLICATION DATA

Xenobiotics : new research / [edited by] Saul F. Castaneda and Mauro L. Emerson.
p. cm.
Includes index.
ISBN 978-1-61942-616-0 (hardcover)
1. Xenobiotics. I. Castaneda, Saul F. II. Emerson, Mauro L.
QP529.X476 2011
616.97'071--dc23
2011050992

Published by Nova Science Publishers, Inc. † New York

CONTENTS

PREFACE

A xenobiotic is a chemical which is found in an organism but which is not normally produced or expected to be present in it. Specifically, drugs such as antibiotics are xenobiotics in humans because the human body does not produce them itself. In this new book, the authors present current research on xenobiotics including the potential effects of toxic agents on immune system function; medical strategies to prevent adverse effects of PAH-like anthropogenic xenobiotics; organophosphorus pesticides as dangerous xenobiotics for aquatic environments and phytoremediation for removal of organic xenobiotics from water.

Chapter 1 - To study the potential effects of toxic agents on immune system function and/or integrity, methods that can be validated in animal models and which provide results capable of being extrapolated to human health need to be developed. This damage can also be evaluated in key species within trophic webs or in those that are biologically important per se. Absence of general agreement as to the biomarkers to be used in the field of Immunotoxicity reveals the need for definite protocols associated with the complexities of immune response. Three types of strategies are described; rather than being mutually exclusive, they are parts of an integral whole and their results run the gamut from the simple to the complex. The basic type I strategies includes evaluations of lymphoid cells and related blood chemistry. The extended type I strategies comprises the function of subpopulations involved in cellular and humoral response. Type II includes assays for T cell-dependent and independent antigens, B cells, cellular immunoreactivity and, most of all, co-exposure to infectious contagious agents or tumoral cells. The metabolic type III and histopathologic type III strategies have to do with immune system organs. Nevertheless, current evidence indicates that immune system damage may often be modulated by changes associated with the bioactivation of toxic agents in non lymphoid organs, which can alter immune system function at the pre- and post-transcriptional level.

Chapter 2 - Cytochromes P450 1A sub-family (CYP1A1 and CYP1A2) are well-known metabolizers of anthropogenic compounds such as polycyclic aromatic hydrocarbons (PAHs) and arylamines. They catalyze all metabolic reactions occurring with PAHs in the organism including the ones resulting in the formation of carcinogenic, mutagenic and teratogenic substances. PAH in their intact, exogenous form usually do not produce adverse effects on the organism (except rare cases of acute poisoning with extremely high doses), however, their metabolites are able to bind and damage macromolecules in the cells. PAHs characterized by specific physical and chemical properties: they are hydrophobic, planar molecules with the size of approximately 6.8 x 13.7 Å. In organisms, PAH activate expression of CYP1A and serve as their substrates. PAH-like inducers of CYP1A are called "classic" inducers. They increase CYP1A activity hundreds fold, undergo metabolic activation and, afterwards, become able to promote the development of dangerous diseases including chemically-induced cancer.

Recent studies demonstrate an increasing number of non-PAH-like CYP1A inducers, which have different physical and chemical properties. These substances include endogenous compounds and food components, such as indoles, flavonoids, vitamins, and some others. They are so-called "weak" or "non-classical" CYP1A inducers and they increase the enzyme activity not more than several times. This mild activation of CYP1A by naturally-occuring substances probably has a physiological function and is not dangerous for organisms.

At least some “weak” CYP1A inducers are able to inhibit the effect of "classic" inducers such as 2,3,7,8-Tetrachlorodibenzodioxin (TCDD) or benzo(a)pyrene in the case of combined administration. Since classic inducers are metabolized by CYP1A to reactive intermediates able to cause chemically-induced cancer and other diseases, the suppression of CYP1A activity might be a useful tool for their prevention and/or management. Thus, detailed understanding of molecular mechanisms underlying this phenomenon is required. Further investigation of “weak” CYP1A inducers might result in the development of new medical strategies to prevent or fight adverse effects of PAH-like anthropogenic xenobiotics.

Chapter 3 - Organophosphorus pesticides (OP) are dangerous xenobiotics for aquatic environments mainly because they can interact with all links of the food web inducing bioaccumulation and bioconcentration in organisms. In addition, they have an influence on the enzymes of the cholinergic system (acetylcholinesterase and pseudocholinesterase) of the organisms blocking their catalytic site and causing an excess of excitation of receptors for acetylcholine accumulation. The biomarkers, such as the evaluation of acetylcholinesterase (AChE) inhibition, provide an indication of the pollution level of the environment and are indicators of the ecotoxicological risk for exposed organisms. As small invertebrates are a fundamental link in the food web, the ecotoxicological risk evaluated on these organisms with the biomarker approach can be used as an early evidence of ecosystem damage. In this research copepods collected in the splashpools of the eastern coast of the Ligurian Sea and maintained in the laboratory were utilized as test-organisms. Aim of this work was to evaluate in copepods *Tigriopus fulvus* the effect of the exposition to the organophosphorus pesticide Malathion (Pestanal®) on the activity of AChE.

Chapter 4 - Resurgence in the use of soil-applied residual herbicides to augment performance of failing post-emergence herbicides has predictably reignited concerns over potential offsite movement, carryover damage onsite, or potential herbicide failure due to accelerated degradation. Many of the key processes in herbicide fate are relatively well-described, however, the bulk of our knowledge of herbicide transformation in soil is based on assumed aerobic conditions, which leaves gaps in our understanding of events taking place during transient saturation. Many areas of agricultural production are vulnerable to periodic flooding, which results in slower O_2 replenishment, and thus promotes local anoxia. Variation in water content through its extremes modulates the bioavailability of substrates to microorganisms, as well as the dominant types of organisms and their associated activities (due to fluctuation of redox regime). Most information about anaerobic processes of herbicide degradation in soil has been derived from experiments performed under long-term submersion, however some studies have demonstrated significant impact of even transient soil saturation on herbicide degradation. A thorough analysis of available data is needed not only to address the current frequency of soil saturation events, but also anticipated changes in water regime as global climates shift. For example, in the American Midwest, projected changes in rainfall patterns are expected to have profound influence on soil water status and variability. Herein, we review literature available on herbicide fate processes as a function of soil water regime, including transient flooding. Examples are presented of herbicides undergoing degradation under denitrifying and iron-reducing conditions, which are most likely to be encountered under transient flooding. New findings are presented for reductive dehalogenation and potential for this process under transient flooding. Also described are water effects on the ecology and activities of herbicide-degrading microorganisms, as well as recent advancements in methodology available to address unanswered research questions in this area.

Chapter 5 - Heavy metals, anthropogenic toxicants, can penetrate into the human organism in tiny amounts through food and water and then accumulate, promoting oppression of mono-oxygenase systems of a liver and possesses pro-oxidative and mutagen activity In this paper, pathological disorders in liver due to heavy metals effects and their treatment have been investigated. The obtained data has confirmed the fact that in activation and deactivation of the mutagens the big role is played by free radicals, condition MOS and antioxidative organism systems. It was shown that the course of the entero-sorption therapy by a citric pectin sorbent in a combination with antioxidative phyto-preparation provides reducing of intensity of the generated pathological variations.

Chapter 6 - Pollution by persistent organic pollutants (pesticides, pharmaceuticals, petroleum hydrocarbons, PAHs, PCBs, etc.) is an environmental problem that is recognized worldwide. In order to address this problem, cost effective technologies have been developed and evaluated for the decontamination of soil and water resources. Phytoremediation is a promising technology that uses plants and the associated rhizosphere microorganisms to remove, transform/detoxify, or accumulate organic and inorganic pollutants present in soils, sediments, surface or ground water, wastewater, and even the atmosphere. In fact, as a result of their sedentary nature, plants have evolved diverse abilities for dealing with toxic compounds in their environment. They, therefore, possess a variety of pollutant attenuation mechanisms that makes their use in remediating contaminated land and water more feasible than physical and chemical remediation. Currently, phytoremediation is used for treating many classes of organic xenobiotics including petroleum hydrocarbons, chlorinated solvents, polycyclic aromatic hydrocarbons, pesticides, explosives, pharmaceutical compounds and their metabolites, and it involves several decontamination mechanisms. There are several different types of phytotechnologies such as, for instance, treatment constructed wetlands. The aim of this work is to present a review on the application of phytoremediation technologies for water decontamination from persistent organic pollutants, with special emphasis focused on the removal of a class of emergent pollutants that has recently been receiving a lot of attention, the pharmaceutically active compounds. Within the realm of phytotechnologies, constructed wetlands for wastewater treatment deserve a special focus as these systems have been used with success for the removal of several different types of organic xenobiotics.

Chapter 7 - It is widely accepted that the current and planned increase in commercial development of nanotechnology will lead to pronounced releases of nanomaterials (NM) in the environment. In this study we aim to evaluate the toxicity of silver nanoparticles and some chlorinated phenol compounds by using a common sludge bacterium, Pseudomonas putida (originally isolated from activated sludge) as biosensor in bioluminescence assays. The results of the toxicity testing were expressed as IC50 values which represents the amount of toxicants required to reduce light output by 50% and calculated using a statistical program that was developed in-house. The bacterium carrying a stable chromosomal copy of the lux operon (luxCDABE) was able to detect toxicity of ionic and particulate silver over short term incubations ranging from 30-240 min. The IC50 values obtained at different time intervals showed that highest toxicity (lowest IC50) was obtained after 90 min incubation for all toxicants and this is considered the optimum incubation for testing. The data show that ionic silver is most toxic followed by nanosilver particles with microsilver particles being least toxic. Release of nanomaterials is likely to have an effect on the activated sludge process as indicated by this study using a common sludge bacterium involved in biodegradation of organic wastes. Among the chlorinated phenol compounds, 3,5 dichlorophenol showed the highest toxicity and phenol being the least toxic. Among the hydroxylated compounds tested, benzoquinone showed to be the most toxic compound. Understanding the fate and transport of phenolic compounds and transformation products in removal treatment plants is relevant in evaluating the impact of discharge in the environment and in developing a program for pollution control. Our results demonstrate that the use of a bacterial biosensor as P. putida BS566::luxCDABE, native from a highly polluted environment, provides a robust, early warning system of acute toxicity which could lead to process failure. This strain is suitable for toxicity monitoring in a highly polluted industrial waste water treatment streams and it has the potential to inform on upstream process changes prior to their impacting upon the biological remediation section.

In: Xenobiotics: New Research
Editors: Saul F. Castaneda and Mauro L. Emerson
ISBN: 978-1-61942-616-0

Chapter 1

PROTOCOLS FOR THE STUDY OF IMMUNOTOXICITY: A REVIEW

M. Lilia Domínguez-López[1], Yolanda Ortega-Ortega[1], Luís A. Jiménez-Zamudio[2], Ethel García-Latorre[1] and Armando Vega-López[3]*

[1]Laboratorio de Inmunoquímica I

[2]Laboratorio de Inmunología Clínica, Departamento de Inmunología, Escuela Nacional de Ciencias Biológicas, Instituto Politécnico Nacional. Carpio y Plan de Ayala s/n, Col. Casco de Santo Tomás, México D.F., Mexico

[3]Laboratorio de Toxicología Ambiental, Departamento de Ingeniería en Sistemas Ambientales, Escuela Nacional de Ciencias Biológicas, Instituto Politécnico Nacional. Av. Wilfrido Massieu s/n, Unidad Profesional Zacatenco, México D.F., México

ABSTRACT

To study the potential effects of toxic agents on immune system function and/or integrity, methods that can be validated in animal models and which provide results capable of being extrapolated to human health need to be developed. This damage can also be evaluated in key species within trophic webs or in those that are biologically important per se. Absence of general agreement as to the biomarkers to be used in the field of Immunotoxicity reveals the need for definite protocols associated with the complexities of immune response. Three types of strategies are described; rather than being mutually exclusive, they are parts of an integral whole and their results run the gamut from the simple to the complex. The basic type I strategies includes evaluations of lymphoid cells and related blood chemistry. The extended type I strategies comprises the function of subpopulations involved in cellular and humoral response. Type II includes assays for T cell-dependent and independent antigens, B cells, cellular immunoreactivity and, most of all, co-exposure to infectious contagious agents or tumoral cells. The metabolic type III and histopathologic type III strategies have to do with immune system

* Corresponding author: Tel: (+52 55) 57296300x52320. Fax (+52 55) 57296300x52301; E-mail address: avegadv@yahoo.com.mx

organs. Nevertheless, current evidence indicates that immune system damage may often be modulated by changes associated with the bioactivation of toxic agents in non lymphoid organs, which can alter immune system function at the pre- and post-transcriptional level.

INTRODUCTION

Exposure to diverse substances of natural or synthetic origin can alter the function and/or integrity of different systems, including the immune system (Bernier *et al.*, 1995; Reynaud and Deschaux 2006; Zinedine *et al.*, 2007). Over 100,000 synthetic chemicals are estimated to exist according to the National Institute for Occupational Safety and Health (NIOSH) of the Centers for Disease Control and Prevention (U.S.DHHS, 1997). On top of this, the large number of both organic and inorganic toxicants of natural origin in which exposure usually takes place in an uncontrolled manner must be considered. Natural resource use and environmental accidents are the most common routes of contact with these toxicants. According to the annual report of the US Agency for Toxic Substances and Disease Registry (ATSDR), 275 substances are extremely hazardous to both ecosystems and human health (ATSDR, 2008). The Comprehensive Environmental Response, Compensation, and Liability Act (CERCLA) has estimated, with the use of algorithms, that at least 859 substances are candidates for inclusion in its Priority List of Hazardous Substances, although toxicity profiles for these are not available (www.atsdr.cdc.gov/pdns/). It should be pointed out that these criteria have been established mostly on the basis of systemic toxicity, but a large number of studies are still needed on their effects on the immune system. One of the areas of fastest advance in terms of knowledge within the biomedical sciences is Immunology. However, there are important information shortages, particularly with regard to the impact of toxicants on the immune system of numerous zoological groups. Immunotoxicology, which is a subdiscipline of Immunology or Toxicology depending on the standpoint used, is the science providing proof of this damage. However, there is a lack of information on both problem diagnosis and research strategies on the matter.

Immunosuppression, nonspecific immunostimulation, hypersensitivity and autoimmunity are the most common types of response evaluated in immunotoxicity studies (Descotes, 2006). Reduction in the number of immunocompetent cells, changes in the function of these cells, and lymphocyte selection and differentiation can favor the development of numerous diseases (Pallardy *et al.*, 1999). However, in epidemiological and clinical studies confusing factors may be present, leading usually to erroneous interpretations (Vos and van Loveren, 1998). In part this is due to a lack of consensus as to the capacity of screening protocols to reflect the damage induced by different toxicants on the immune system (Baken *et al.*, 2007; de Jong and van Loveren, 2007; Ladics, 2007) as well as to absence of information on the matter. This review is intended to extend current knowledge on the impact of toxicants on immune system integrity and/or function.

STRATEGIES FOR THE STUDY OF TOXICANT IMPACT ON THE IMMUNE SYSTEM

Research strategies in the field of immunotoxicology can be proposed without ruling out the complex character of immune response and the numerous aspects requiring discussion in toxicological studies. These strategies can at least be categorized based on the complexity of the biomarkers used in immunotoxicology as well as experimental design. The first category evaluates immune system function by exposing the test organism to immunotoxicants. The second includes, in addition to this, co-exposure to pathogenic microorganisms or infectious agents, which is known as immunization or antigenic challenge (WHO, 1986). The third category includes histopathological and metabolic changes to immune system organs in addition to mortality or morbidity studies. Even congenital malformations in immune system organs and marked predisposition to maternal infections during gestation can be evaluated if an adequate study model is used. The first two strategies should be carried out using sub lethal concentrations or doses, and their duration goes from short-term to sub chronic exposure levels. The third strategy may be short-term or may reach sub chronic, chronic and generational (F_1 and F_2) exposure levels.

Basic strategies: These include cellular evaluation and assessment of hematologic and biochemical parameters such as:

- Changes in peripheral blood mononuclear cell count.
- Alterations in lymphocyte populations, such as lymphocytosis, lymphopenias and eosinophilia.
- Clinical chemistry biomarkers including serum albumin, the albumin/globulin (A/G) ratio, and transaminases.

Expanded basic strategies: Besides the basic biomarkers mentioned above, these include:

- Flow cytometry analysis of lymphocyte subpopulations, such as B lymphocytes, T lymphocytes, and their subpopulations: CD4+ (Th1 and Th2) and CD8+ (Tc1 and Tc2). Alterations in the relative proportions of these subpopulations (e.g. CD4+/CD8+) may indicate immunotoxicity. Serum levels of α, β, and γ globulin and the immunoglobulins (IgG, IgM, and IgA) should be analyzed by electrophoretic methods. Evaluation of complement molecules such as C3. Immunodetection of cytokines, antibodies, and bactericidal activity.
- Quantification of antibodies including antinuclear, antimitochondrial and antiparietal cell antibodies. Immunotoxic properties can be attributed to the substance studied if these changes are significant with respect to controls in a controlled experimental scheme. In the case of pharmaceuticals such as isoniazid or hydralazine, production of auto-antibodies is due to formation of neoantigens by metabolites of the pharmaceutical agent and complement molecules (Sim, 1989).
- Functional evaluation *in vitro* of certain lymphoid cell lineages: NK cell activity can be estimated by chromium release assay or biological challenge tests, both of which estimate their capacity to destroy cancerous or virus-infected cells.

- Mitogen-induced B and T-cell stimulation: Certain plant lectins and lipopolysaccharides can induce blastogenesis and DNA synthesis in immune system mononuclear cells from peripheral blood or spleen-derived cell suspensions. *Ex vitro* tests using phytohemagglutinin or concanavalin A stimulate T-cell proliferation, while bacterial lipopolysaccharides do so in B cells. The lectin of pokeweed (*Phytolacca americana*), which is an activator of both B and T cells, should receive special mention. Similarly, T cells may show response to allogeneic cells.
- To evaluate mitogen-induced lymphoproliferation, assays that incorporate radioactive elements such as tritiated thymidine are used. However, since these tests depend on the facilities of the laboratory for handling these elements, simpler strategies with fewer technical restrictions are often employed, such as bromodeoxyuridine incorporation or evaluation of mitochondrial activity through MTT [3-(4,5-dimethyl-2-thiazolyl)-2,5-diphenyl-2H-tetrazolium bromide] metabolism. Significant elevations or reductions in this activity may reflect potential risk from exposure to immunotoxicants.
- Phagocytic activity: This strategy is based on the capacity of macrophages to ingest particles such as microscopic plastic balls or iron shavings. However, the best results are obtained with yeasts, either opsonized with specific immunoglobulins or complement, or unopsonized. These assays can be made on peripheral blood cells or cell suspensions from lymphoid organs such as the spleen. Analysis can also be made of the respiratory burst in macrophages by measuring superoxide anion production or lysosomal activity.

Co-exposure strategy: Its development requires, in addition to exposure to the immunotoxicant, certain biological challenge tests or co-exposure to these infectious-contagious agents in order to evaluate potential alterations in immune system function which may target a particular cell type. Exposure to the immunotoxicant requires a well-defined experimental design, justifying test duration and the dose or concentration used. Separate evaluation of immunotoxicant-induced effects and biological challenge tests is essential, as is the subsequent determination of damage to immune system integrity and/or function induced by co-exposure. Exposure to the immunotoxicant usually precedes exposure to the challenge, although the opposite cannot be ruled out. Justification in this case is based on existence of synergetic, antagonistic, summation or potentiation phenomena. In addition to the biomarkers used in the expanded basic strategies, other tests must be performed, including:

- T cell-dependent antigen test: Antibody-forming cell suspensions are commonly used. These are derived from spleen or peripheral blood from immunized animals exposed to immunotoxicants, and are incubated with sheep erythrocytes on microscope slides. If lymphoid lineage function is preserved, small light-colored areas called plaques are formed. A significant change in the number of plaques with respect to controls indicates immunotoxicity. Other T cell-dependent antigens are also used, while horseshoe crab (*Limulus polyphemus*) hemocyanin and sometimes even bovine serum albumin are employed as a challenge prior to treating the animals with the immunotoxicant.

- T cell-independent antigen test: The same cell types as above are used on the animals exposed, but the antigenic challenge is different. In this case the choice is ficoll, a branched chain polysaccharide. Ficoll plus haptens, polyvinylpyrrolidone and bacterial lipopolysaccharides may also be used.
- Human vaccines as a challenge: Animals are first exposed to the toxicant and are subsequently administered human vaccines that are either T lymphocyte-dependent, as in the case of the tetanus toxoid, or B lymphocyte-dependent like the vaccine against *Pneumococcus* spp. Significant alterations in immune response with respect to controls are proof of immunotoxicity.
- Cell-mediated immunoreactivity: Contact sensitizers such as dinitrochlorobenzene applied on the epidermis of an animal pre-exposed to xenobiotics are used. Delayed hypersensitivity is a reliable indicator of cell-mediated immunoreactivity. Besides being cost-effective, this test may be associated with reduced resistance to pathogens or infectious agents.
- Popliteal lymphatic gland assay: In these test small doses of the immunotoxicant are administered subcutaneously by injection in the popliteal fascia. Inflammation of lymphatic glands in this area may be associated with potential risk of induction of autoimmune disorders by the xenobiotic (Pieters and Albers, 1999).
- Test of host resistance to infectious agents: This is one of the most important tests in the field of immunotoxicology and reflects the integral impact on the immune system in animals exposed to xenobiotics. A large number of pathogenic strains characteristic of each of the species under study are used, including bacteria, parasites, fungi, viruses, etc. that are of concern for each type of organism. In this assay, exposing the species to the immunotoxicant first (pre-exposure) and subsequently to the challenge (co-exposure) is recommended (Dean and Thurmond, 1987). When adequate facilities are available, continuous exposure to the immunotoxicant can be carried out. However, with this experimental design, adaptation to or recovery from the immunotoxicant is possible, with consequent underestimation of immune system response. In organisms that are environmentally exposed to mixtures of xenobiotics, it is irresponsible to say that alterations in immune response, such as increased parasitosis or disease, are due to toxicant-induced effects or vice versa. For example, one of the strategies of macrophages and monocytes against parasites, microbes and cancerous or virus-infected cells is the respiratory burst. This phenomenon produces increases in oxidative stress in the organs in which these cellular interactions take place such as the mucosa, spleen, liver, etc., together with chain reactions that can potentially damage other organs. If environmentally exposed specimens are collected and evaluated using typical biomarkers in toxicology – such as oxidative stress – and additionally show high parasitosis, morbidity or mortality, it is almost impossible to say which of the two situations produced the other, or if synergism or potentiation were involved. Potential alternatives are easily noted: Was a toxicant-induced increase in oxidative stress the factor responsible for increased susceptibility of the host? Or did the immune system strategies of the host in response to the pathogen induce this oxidative

stress? Thus, it is essential to have at one's disposal experimental models that are able to reveal the relationships between these responses, since erroneous conclusions are frequently arrived at with this type of casual observation (Wu *et al.*, 2005).

- Test of host resistance to tumoral cells: Contrary to evaluation against infectious agents, in this assay the natural biological barriers of an organism pre-exposed to an immunotoxicant are artificially modified. Tumoral cells are directly inoculated in the specimen and potential tumor development is then monitored. One validated protocol uses the PYB6 sarcoma and B16F10 melanoma cell lines (Murray *et al.*, 1985). For evident reasons, this field has received little study, although this has benefits as well as drawbacks. It is interesting because cell lines are used that are heterologous to the pre-exposed species and this may involve a very pronounced immune response, unlike the case of natural infectious agents in which interrelationships may already have been developed, in particular humoral immunity and the complement system. An outstanding drawback is that in natural conditions these interactions between cancerous cells and the exposed heterologous organism almost never take place.

Strategies of Metabolic Response in Immune System Cells

Immune system organs have very specific metabolic characteristics with respect to the reference organ, which in toxicology is the liver or, in lower organisms, the hepatopancreas. This is the most important organ from the standpoint of biotransformation (Whyte *et al.*, 2000; van der Oost *et al.*, 2003). Diverse mechanisms of immunotoxicity exist and will depend on many variables such as biological, environmental and experimental factors as well as the properties of toxic agents.

The characteristics of hazardous substances are particularly useful for evaluating "nonreactive toxicity", i.e. when the mechanism of toxicity of these substances does not involve participation of the receptors (Blum and Speece, 1990). These properties can be summarized according to quantitative structure-activity relationships (QSARs). The octanol-water partition coefficient (log P) comprises the relative partition of the toxicant into an aqueous (polar) phase and an octanol (apolar) phase as a dynamic simulation of the extracellular medium-lipidic biphase. Solvatochronic parameters (linear solvation energy relationships, LSERs) include four characteristics of toxicants: (i) intrinsic molecular volume, (ii) polarity, and their capacity to function as (iii) hydrogen donors or (iv) hydrogen acceptors (Kamlet *et al.*, 1986). Both log P and LSERs are based on Hansch analysis, in which the physicochemical properties of the toxicants are considered (Blum and Speece, 1990). Molecular connectivity describes molecular topology, in which the valence index provides information on both volume and the electron configuration of the toxon. Its usefulness lies in predicting relationships between bioactivity of the toxicant and its molecular characteristics, which include a balance between valence and non-valence indexes. First- and second-degree equations can in this way be predicted (Kier, 1981).

Table 1. Basic and expanded strategies for the study of Immunotoxicity, some published studies

Inmunotoxic	Biomarker/species	Experimental design /study	Response	Reference
Ag (as nanoparticles)	IL-1B, TNF (R.n)	In vitro	+	Trickler et al., 2010
Al	Lymphoproliferation and phagocytic activity (T.t)	In vitro	—	Cámara-Pellissó et al., 2008
Pb	T-cell response (PHA skin test) C.c.j	In vivio	NS	Nain & Smits, 2011
Cd	Phagocytic activity and T-cell response (PHA skin test) C.c.j	In vivo	—	Nad et al., 2009
Cd	Lymphoproliferation and phagocytic activity (T.t)	In vitro	—	Cámara-Pellissó et al., 2008
Cd	IL-2 and IFNγ (M.m.)	In vitro	+	Pathak & Khandelwal, 2008
Cr^{+6}	Maturation of dendritic cells (H.s)	In vitro/ Cr uptake	+	Burastero et al., 2006
Cu	Leukocyte counts (C.m)	In vivo	+/-	Lugo et al., 2006
Pd, Pt, Rh, Ti, As,	Lymphoproliferation, Phagocytic activity, Cytokines (H.s)	Ex vivo	–	Di Gioacchino et al., 2007
Hg	Phagocytosis (S.p)	In vivo/ in situ	–	Ahmad et al., 2011
Hg (as $HgCl_2$)	Autoimmune hepatitis (M.m)	In vivo	+	Gilbert et al., 2011
Hg	Antinuclear and antinucleolar auto-antibodies (H.s)	Epidemiology/ occupational	+	Gardner et al., 2010
Hg	IL-1β, TNF-α, and IFN-γ	Epidemiology/ occupational	+	Gardner et al., 2010
Hg	Lymphoproliferation and phagocytic activity (T.t)	In vitro	—	Cámara-Pellissó et al., 2008
Hg	Lupus erythematosus (M.m)	In vivo	+	Silbergeld et al., 2005
Hg	Autoimmune diseases (H.s)	Epidemiology/ Trophic	+	Bernier et al., 1995
Hg	Proinflammatory cytokines (H.s)	Epidemiology/ Trophic	+	Bernier et al., 1995
Ni	Hypersensitivity type I and IV T-cell mediated	Epidemiology/ occupational and non-occupational	+	Hostynek, 2006
Inmunotoxic	Biomarker/species	Experimental design /study	Response	Reference

Table 1. Continued

Inmunotoxic	Biomarker/species	Experimental design /study	Response	Reference
Pb	Proportion of CD4+/CD8+ cells (H.s)	Epidemiology/ occupational	+	García-Lestón et al., 2011
Pb	Proportion of CD8+ cells (H.s)	Epidemiology/ occupational and non-occupational	-	García-Lestón et al., 2011
Pb	TLR-3 expression (C.c.j)	In vivo	+	Nain & Smits, 2011
Pb	Lymphoproliferation (T.t)	In vitro	—	Cámara-Pellissó et al., 2008
Pb	Myeloid suppressor cells count	In vitro	+	Farrer et al., 2008
Pb	Autoimmune diseases (H.s)	Epidemiology/ Trophic	+	Bernier et al., 1995
Pb	Proinflammatory cytokines (H.s)	Epidemiology/ Trophic	+	Bernier et al., 1995
Pb	TNF-α m-RNA	In vivo	+	Khan et al., 2011
Pb	TNF-α	In vivo	+	
Cd	Autoimmune diseases (H.s)	Epidemiology/ Trophic	+	Bernier et al., 1995
Cd	Proinflammatory cytokines (H.s)	Epidemiology/ Trophic	+	Bernier et al., 1995
Cd	Ig's production (R.n)	In vivo	+	Descotes, 1992
Cd	Lymphoproliferation (R.n)	Ex vivo	–	Descotes, 1992
Cd	Phagocytic activity (R.n)	Ex vivo	–	Descotes, 1992
Cd	NKT-cell activity (R.n)	Ex vivo	–	Descotes, 1992
Zn	Proliferation of B-cell (P.v)	In vitro	+	Frouin et al., 2010
Zn	Haemocytes, phagocytic activity (H.t.)	In vitro	–	Mottin et al., 2010
Heavy metals mixtures	Proportion of CD3+ and CD4+ cells (H.s)	Epidemiology/occupational and non-occupational	–	Coelho et al., 2011
Heavy metals mixtures	Proportion of CD16/56+ cells (H.s)	Epidemiology/occupational and non-occupational	+	Coelho et al., 2011
As, Se, Va, Ag, Fe	Proliferation of B-cell line (P.v)	In vitro	–	Frouin et al., 2010
As, Se, Va, Zn	Phagocytic activity (P.v)	In vitro	–	Frouin et al., 2010
Organophosphorus pesticides	NK activity (R.n)	Epidemiology	+	Li et al., 2002
Organophosphorus	Cytokines (H.s)	Epidemiology	–	Li et al., 2002;

pesticides				Li y Kawada 2006
Organophosphorus pesticides	Inhibition of granzimes (H.s)	Epidemiology	+	Li et al., 2002
Organophosphorus pesticides	Inhibition of perforins (H.s)	Epidemiology	+	Li et al., 2002
Organophosphorus pesticides	Degranulation of NK cells (H.s)	In vitro	+	Li et al., 2005
Organophosphorus pesticides	Apoptosis and necrosis of PBMCs (H.s)	Epidemiology	+	Das et al., 2006
Organophosphorus pesticides	Humoral response (H.s)	Epidemiology	–	Das et al., 2006
Organophosphorus pesticides	Cytokines Th1/Th2	Epidemiology	+	Li & Kawada 2006
Organophosphorus pesticides	Decrease of CD5+	Epidemiology	+	Li & Kawada 2006
Organophosphorus pesticides	Increase of CD26+	Epidemiology	+	Li & Kawada 2006
Organophosphorus pesticides	Autoantibody production	Epidemiology	+	Li & Kawada 2006
Benzo[a]pyrene	Proliferation of B-cell line (P.v)	In vitro	–	Frouin et al., 2010
Benzo[a]pyrene	Phagocytic activity (P.v)	In vitro	–	Frouin et al., 2010
Benzo[a]pyrene	Macrophage expression of CXCR5, GPR35, and RASAL1 (H.s)	In vitro	+	Sparfel et al., 2010
Benzo[a]pyrene	Lymphoproliferation (M.m)	In vivo	–	Schellenberger et al., 2009
Methyl isocyanate	Proinflammatory cytokines (H.s)	In vitro	+	Mishra et al., 2008
Asphalt	IgM production (M.m)	In vivo	–	Anderson et al., 2008
HAPs mixture	Lymphoproliferation (H.s)	Ex vivo	–	Davila et al., 1995
PCBs	Ig's production (H.s)	Epidemiology/ maternal and early postnatal	NS	Jusko et al., 2011
PCB 153	Splenic lymphoproliferation (L.m)	In vivo	–	Duffy-Whritenour et al., 2010
Aroclor 1248	T-cell response (PHA) A.n	In vivo	+	Iwanowicz et al., 2009
PCB mono-ortho	Lymphoproliferation (PHA, ConcA, PWM) H.g	In vitro	–	Sørmo et al., 2009
PCB 126	B-cell response (G.d)	In vivo	–	Lavoie et al., 2007

Table 1. Continued

Inmunotoxic	Biomarker/species	Experimental design /study	Response	Reference
PCB 126	T-cell response (PHA) G.d	In vivo	NS	Lavoie et al., 2007
PCB 126 and 77	B-cell response (G.d)	In vivo	–	Lavoie & Grasman, 2007
PCB 126 and 77	T-cell response (PHA) G.d	In vivo	NS	Lavoie & Grasman, 2007
PCBs	Immunotoxicity (P.v)	In situ	+	
PCBs	Phagocytic activity (M.s.)	In vivo	+	Zelikoff et al., 2000.
PBDEs	Neutrophils count (M.v)	In situ	+	Martin et al., 2007
PBDEs	Lymphocytes count (M.v)	In situ	–	Martin et al., 2007
PCBs, PCDFs, PCDDs	NK-cell activity (P.v)	Trophic	+	Ross et al., 1996
PCBs, PCDFs, PCDDs	Lymphoproliferation (P.v.)	Ex vivo	–	Ross et al., 1996
PBDE	Splenocytes count (M.m)	In vivo/ Gestational	–	Gill et al., 2004
Aflatoxine	Lymphoproliferation and phagocytic activity (several spp.)	In vivo/ Trophic	–	Bondy & Pestka, 2000
Gliotoxine	Lymphoproliferation (R.n)	In vitro	–	Bondy & Pestka, 2000
Ocratoxine	Lymphoproliferation (R.n y M.m)	In vivo/ Trophic	–	Bondy & Pestka, 2000
Fumonisine	Lymphoproliferation (R.n y M.m)	In vivo/ Trophic	–	Bondy & Pestka, 2000
Micotoxines	Lymphoproliferation (B.t)	In vivo/ Trophic	–	Black et al., 1992
Caramel dye III	Lymphocytes count (R.n y M.m)	In vivo/ Trophic	–	Houben & Penninks, 1994
Halotane	Eosinophilia, autoantibody, hepatitis immunoallergic (H.s)	In vivo/ Clinic	+	Dansette et al., 1998.
Thienyl acid	Eosinophilia, autoantibody, hepatitis immunoallergic (H.s)	In vivo/ Clinic	+	Dansette et al., 1998.

Dihydralazine	Eosinophilia, autoantibody, hepatitis immunoallergic (H.s)	In vivo/ Clinic	+	Dansette et al., 1998.
Anticonvulsants	Eosinophilia, autoantibody, hepatitis immunoallergic (H.s)	In vivo/ Clinic	+	Dansette et al., 1998.
Corticoesteroids	Immunosuppression (H.s)	In vivo/ Clinic	+	Pruett et al., 1993; Bálint & Gergely, 1996
Asbest	Immunosuppression (H.s)	Epidemiology	+	Luster & Rosenthal, 1993
Benzene	Immunosuppression (H.s)	Epidemiology	+	Luster & Rosenthal, 1993
Metotrexate	Immunosuppression (H.s)	In vivo/ Clinic	+	Bálint & Gergely, 1996
Hydralazine	Lupus erythematosus (H.s)	In vivo/ Clinic	+	Sim, 1989
Isoniazide	Lupus erythematosus (H.s)	In vivo/ Clinic	+	Sim, 1989
Inmunotoxic	Biomarker/species	Experimental design /study	Response	Reference
Procainamide	Lupus erythematosus (H.s)	In vivo/ Clinic	+	Sim,1989
Penicilamine	Lupus erythematosus (H.s)	In vivo/ Clinic	+	Sim, 1989

+ Increase. – Decrease. NS= No significant. In situ: Free ranging specimens. H.s= *Homo sapiens*. R.n= *Rattus norvegicus*. M.m= *Mus musculus*. M.s.=*Micropterus salmoides*. P.v.= *Phoca vitulina* B.t= *Bus taurus*. S.p.= *Scrobicularia plana*. H.t= *Haliotis tuberculata*. C.m= *Colossoma macropomum*. C.c.j= *Coturnix coturnix japonica*. T.t= *Tursiops truncates*. L.m= *Lepomis macrochirus*. A.n= *Ameiurus nebulosus*. H.g= *Halichoerus grypus*. G.d= *Gallus domesticus*. M.v=*Mustela vison*.

Length of exposure and test concentration or dose is among the most important experimental conditions. As regards the former, the life cycle of the test organism or the purpose of the experiment should be taken into consideration. When mortality or immobility of 50% of the organisms exposed is sought, exposure will be short-term and assays are called "acute" (USDHHS, 1997). Duration is usually 24-48 h in the case of invertebrate organisms and 96 h when dealing with vertebrates (/www.epa.gov/waterscience/methods/wet/disk2/). There is no general consensus, but many authors use the term "sub acute assays" to refer to tests in which the period of exposure is comparatively longer than in acute assays but shorter than in sub chronic assays, which comprise 1/3 to 2/3 of the life cycle of the organism. Chronic assays must cover at least 2/3 or up to 3/3 of the life cycle of the specimen (USDHHS, 1997). Organisms exposed in their natural environment, where neither length of exposure nor actual fluctuations in environmental levels of the toxicant can be determined during the life cycle of the specimen, can only be termed "environmentally exposed organisms".

Table 2. Co-exposure strategy for the study of Immunotoxicity, some published studies

Inmunotoxic	Biomarker/challenge/ species	Experimental design	Response	Reference
V^{+5}	Bacterial resistance (R.n)	In vivo	—	Cohen et al., 2010
Cr^{+6}	Bacterial resistance (R.n)	In vivo	—	Cohen et al., 2010
Hg	Viral resistance (coxsackievirus B3) M.m.	In vivo	—	Frisk et al., 2008
Ni	Viral and bacterial resistance (recurrent herpes labialis, urinary tract infections, genital candidiasis, upper respiratory tract infections) H.s	Epidemiology/Ni-hypersensitivity	—	Rosato et al., 2009
Ni	T-cell mediated hypersensitivity (H.s.)	Epidemiologic	+	Hostýnek, 2002; 2006
Pb	Bacterial resistance (*E. coli*) C.c.j	In vivo	+	Nain & Smits, 2011
Pb	B-cell response (Newcastle vaccine) C.c.j	In vivo	NS	Nain & Smits, 2011
Pb	Host resistance (S) H.s	Epidemiologic	+	Luebke et al., 2006
TCDD	Host resistance (S) R.n	In vivo	+	Luebke et al., 2006
TBTO	Host resistance (S) R.n	In vivo	+	Luebke et al., 2006
DES	Host resistance (S) R.n	In vivo	+	Luebke et al., 2006
Diazepam	Host resistance (S) R.n	In vivo	+	Luebke et al., 2006
Hg	Host resistance (S) H.s	Epidemiologic	—	Moszczyński, 1999
Hg	Host resistance (cancer cells) H.s	Epidemiologic	—	Moszczyński, 1999
Hg	T-cell mediated	Epidemiologic	+/—	Moszczyński,

	hypersensitivity (S) H.s			1999
Hg, Pb, Cd	Host resistance (S) H.s	Epidemiologic / Trophic	+	Bernier et al., 1995
Cd	Host resistance (S) R.n	In vivo	+	Descotes, 1992
Retene (alkyl PAH associated)	Ig's synthesis (*Aeromonas salmonicida*) O.m	In vivo	+	Hogan et al., 2010
Benzo[a]pyrene	Lymphoproliferation (B[a]P-diphtheria toxoid conjugate vaccine) M.m	In vivo	+	Schellenberger et al., 2009
Benzo[a]pyrene	Innate immunity and B-cell response (B[a]P-diphtheria toxoid conjugate vaccine) M.m	In vivo	+	Schellenberger et al., 2009
PAHs mixture	B-cell response (marine bacteria) F.h	In situ	—	Frederick et al., 2007
PAHs mixture	Innate immunity (marine bacteria) F.h	In situ	+	Frederick et al., 2007
Micotoxines	Host resistance (S) B.t	Trophic	+	Black et al., 1992
PCBs	B-cell response (diphtheria and tetanus toxoids vaccines) H.s	Epidemiology	—	Heilmann et al., 2010
Aroclor 1248	Bacterial resistance and B-cell response (*Edwardsiella ictaluri*) A.n	In vivo	–	Iwanowicz et al., 2009
PCB's, PCDF's, PCDD's	Host resistance (S) P.v	Trophic	+	van Loveren et al., 2000
PCBs, PCDFs, PCDDs	T-cell mediated hypersensitivity (S) P.v	Ex vivo	+	Ross et al., 1996
PCBs	Host resistance (S) H.s	Epidemiologic/ Trophic	+	Tryphonas, 1995
Cigarette smoke	T-cell mediated hypersensitivity (S) H.s	Epidemiologic / Gestational	+	Selgrade, 2007
As	T-cell mediated hypersensitivity (S) H.s	Epidemiologic / Gestational	+	Selgrade, 2007
Colour additive caramel III	Host resistance (S) R.n, M.m	In vivo/ Trophic	+	Houben & Penninks, 1994

Table 2. Continued

Inmunotoxic	Biomarker/challenge/ species	Experimental design	Response	Reference
Molecular weight compounds	Dendritic cells, T cell and basophils reactivity (S)	In vivo	+	Merk et al., 2001.
Isocyanates	Cellular immunity (S) H.s.	Epidemiologic	+	Luster & Rosenthal, 1993
Anhydrides	Cellular immunity (S) H.s.	Epidemiologic	+	Luster & Rosenthal, 1993

+ Increase. – Decrease NS: No significant change S: varied challenges. In situ: Free ranging specimens. H.s= Homo sapiens. R.n= Rattus norvegicus. B.s= Bus taurus. P.v.= Phoca vitulina. C.c.j= Coturnix coturnix japonica. O.m= Oncorhynchus mykiss. A.n= Ameiurus nebulosus.

As regards concentration or dose, there are ranges inducing mortality or immobility and in this case the tests are called "lethal assays". The term used to refer to these models is meant to express the magnitude of the biological response associated with toxicant amounts. The dose at which 50% mortality is expected in animals exposed is the LD_{50} or lethal dose fifty, and can be calculated by the Probit method or, in its absence; rough estimates can be obtained using the empirical Probit or semi-log methods. Based on these calculations, related percentage values such as the LD_1, LD_{10}, LD_{30} and LD_{99} can be derived. If the test organism is administered the toxicant directly the correct term to use is "dose", but when this substance is measured out into the environment it is called "lethal concentration" (e.g. LC_{50}). Mortality or immobility is discrete variables requiring statistical tests such as χ^2 to confirm the validity of the predictions of these experimental models. LD_0 or LC_0 is the quantity of toxicant considered to induce no mortality or immobility in any of the organisms. However, due to uncertainty as to its upper and lower limits, it cannot be estimated by the Probit method. Use of the semi-log method may thus be advisable for this purpose, although it should be taken into account that this method derives the dose or concentration based on mortality, unlike the Probit method which uses the opposite approach (USDHHS, 1997). Empirical models have been used to find toxicity ratios for estimating the lethal dose zero or lethal concentration zero (LD_0 or $LC_0 \approx 0.15 * LD_{50}$ or LC_{50}, respectively) as well as the maximum allowed concentration ($MAC \approx 0.0013 * LD_{50}$ or LC_{50}) (Jörgensen, 1990). Emphasis is laid on these amounts which neither kill nor immobilize because of their relation to sub lethal assays. The latter usually evaluate biormarkers, which can broadly be defined as quantifiable alterations in biological response. Their purpose is to predict exposure or susceptibility to toxicants, or the damage induced by these (WHO, 1993; Peakall and Shugart, 1994; van der Oost et al., 2003). Sub lethal assay duration is related to the goals of the study and ranges from short-term to chronic exposure levels.

The toxicity of a given substance is influenced by processes such as absorption, distribution, biotransformation and excretion (Repetto, 1997). However, the interpretation of toxicity is a complex task since it depends on extremely important biological responses including initial and maximum induction, adaptation and recovery, which must be seen as an integral process. If these responses are not taken into account, erroneous conclusions with false positives or negatives are likely to be arrived at. Wu *et al.* (2005) found, after an extensive review, that toxic response occurs in different stages. The latency period takes place when the toxicant enters the organism and interacts specifically with its receptors or nonspecifically with different cell components. This period depends on actual toxicant amounts and the time elapsed prior to the occurrence of any biological response. Maximum induction takes place when receptors or target biomolecules become saturated or come into balance with the toxicant(s) in question. However, maximum induction may decline or even reach basal levels if exposure is prolonged. This moment is known as adaptation. Once the toxicant-induced stimulus stops, the toxicant-receptor or toxon-biomolecule complexes that have formed begin to dissociate, and initial recovery takes place. Finally, these stimuli decline below the threshold effect level and the organism exposed goes into full recovery when the damage induced does not alter homeostasis in the organism. The kinetics of damage induction depends on the species studied as well as the xenobiotic.

Taking these stages into account, diverse patterns of toxic response have been determined: (i) *Slow induction followed by adaptation.* This is characterized by a prolonged latency period and the magnitude of the response is not significant with respect to controls. It also depends on the sex of the specimen and affinity of the toxicant for its receptor (Vega-López et al., 2007; 2009). In environmental monitoring, this type of response is unimportant since toxicant concentrations are likely to decline before eliciting maximum induction (Wu *et al.*, 2005). (ii) *Rapid induction followed by adaptation.* The latency period is very short, but maximum induction reverts rapidly to basal levels. Although this response may seem useful for environmental monitoring because it is dose or concentration dependent, it does not provide any information on response over time (Wu *et al.*, 2005). It has been found particularly in females of different species (Vega-López et al., 2007; 2008a). This pattern is usually associated with false positives or negatives. (iii) *Slow induction followed by rapid recovery.* Contrary to the case of pattern (i), the affinity of the toxicant for its receptor is labile, permitting rapid recovery. Fluctuations in environmental levels of the toxicant cannot be evaluated with this type of response (Wu *et al.*, 2005). (iv) *Slow induction followed by slow recovery:* This is the characteristic pattern in situations where contamination levels are relatively stable. However, if fluctuations in levels exist, the response may be considered a false negative or positive due to the pattern of induction. (v) *Rapid induction followed by rapid recovery:* This type of response is very sensitive to environmental fluctuations in contamination levels, but for monitoring to be successful strict control of the length of exposure is necessary (Wu *et al.*, 2005) and its predictive power may be similar to that of evaluation of toxicant concentration in the environment. (vi) *Rapid induction followed by slow recovery:* This type of response may be considered an ideal biomarker (Wu *et al.*, 2005; Vega-López *et al.*, 2009). Rapid induction permits the efficient detection of fluctuations in toxicant concentrations, while prolonged recovery ensures reliability of the response due to quantitative and temporal integration estimation (Wu *et al.*, 2005). A major consideration is that at a particular moment the cumulative potential effects of toxicants or their mixtures may reach threshold levels of damage. It is therefore necessary to have a set of biomarkers at one's disposal. In addition to specific biomarkers associated with certain types of toxons (Whyte *et al.*, 2000), evaluation of broad-range responses such as oxidative stress is recommended (Hermes-Lima, 2004; Vega-López *et al.*, 2007; 2008b; 2009).

Table 3. Strategies of metabolic response in immune system cells and histopathological strategies for the study of Immunotoxicity, some published studies

Inmunotoxic	Biomarker/target/species	Experimental design	Response	Reference
As	G(2)/M phase (lymphoma B-cell line) P.v.	In vitro	—	Frouin et al., 2010
Cd	ROS	In vitro, in vivo, ex vivo	+	Liu et al., 2009
Ni	O_2• (haemocytes) S.s	In vivo	+	Vijayavel et al., 2009
Pb	LPO (haemocytes) S.p.	In situ	+	Ahmad et al., 2011
Pb	NOS (Myeloid suppressor cells) H.s.	In vitro	—	Farrer et al., 2008
Zn	AP, ROS (haemocytes) H.t	In vitro	—	Mottin et al., 2010
Zn	PHL, NSE (haemocytes) H.t	In vitro	+	Mottin et al., 2010
Hg	NOS, Thymulin (plasma) H.s	Occupational exposure	—	Farahat et al., 2009
Hg as MeHg	MT (monocytes) H.s	In vitro	—	Fortier et al., 2008
Hg as MeHg	MT (lymphocytes) H.s	In vitro	+	Fortier et al., 2008
Cd	ROS (T-cells) M.m	In vitro	+	Pathak & Khandelwal, 2008
Cd	GSH (CD4+) M.m	In vitro	—	Pathak & Khandelwal, 2008
Cu, Cr, Pb, Hg	Mast cells infiltration (gills) S.a	In vivo	+	Lauriano et al., 2011
As, Cd, Pb, Hg, Cr, Ni, Mn, Fe mixtures	Lymphoid cell population, atrophic splenic follicles with less follicular activity, and degeneration and necrosis of the lymphoid cells. R.n	In vivo/ subchronic exposure vía drinking water	—	Jadhav et al., 2007
Pd, Pt, Rh	O_2• production	Ex vivo	+	Di Gioacchino et al., 2007
Cs	Splenic irregularities (M.m)	In vivo (gestational)	+	Messiha, 1994
Benzo[a]pyrene	CYP 1A1 activity in	In vivo	+	Schellenberger

	lymphocytes (M.m)			et al., 2009
Benzo[a]pyrene	CYP 1A1 activity in lymphoid cells of the head of the kidney (O.m)	In vivo	+	Nakayama et al., 2008
PAHs mixture	COX-2 activity in lymphoid cells (F.h)	In situ	+	Frederick et al., 2007
2-Chloropropionic acid	ROS and NO production in neutrophil (H.s)	In vitro	+	Aam & Fonnum, 2006
2-Chloropropionic acid	GHS level in neutrophil (H.s)	In vitro	+	Aam & Fonnum, 2006
Retene (alkyl PAH associated)	Increase of B-cell density in spleen and head kidney	In vivo	+	Hogan et al., 2010
Bis(tri-n-butyltin)oxide	Splenic irregularities (M.m)	In vivo	+	Baken et al., 2008
Benzene	No Hodkin lymphoma	Epidemiology	+	Smith et al., 2007
Corticoesteroids	Leukemia and lymphoma (H.s)	In vivo/ clínic	+/–	Bálint y Gergely, 1996
Corticoids	Thymic atrophy (R.n)	In vivo	+	Pruett et al., 1993
PCB 153	ROS in kidney phagocyte (L.m)	In vivo	+	Duffy-Whritenour et al., 2010
PCB 126	Thymus and bursa index (G.d)	In vivo	–	Lavoie et al., 2007
PCB 126 and 77	Thymus and bursa cellularity (G.d)	In vivo	–	Lavoie & Grasman, 2007
PBDEs	Spleen index (M.v)	In vivo	+	Martin et al., 2007
PBDEs	Spleen B-cell hyperplasia (M.v)	In vivo	+	Martin et al., 2007
PCBs, PCDFs, PCDDs	Thymus atrophy (R.n)	In vivo	+	Safe et al., 1989
Tributiltin oxide	Thymus atrophy (R.n)	In vivo	+	Boyer, 1989
Dibutyltin	Thymus atrophy (R.n)	In vivo	+	Boyer, 1989

+ Increase. – Decrease. NS= No significant. In situ: Free ranging specimens. H.s= *Homo sapiens*. R.n= *Rattus norvegicus*. M.m= *Mus musculus*. C.c.= *Cyprinus carpio*. S.p: *Scrobicularia plana* (bivalve). S.a= *Sparus aurata*. H.t= *Haliotis tuberculata* (mollusc) P.v= *Phoca vitulina*. S.s= *Scylla serrata* (mollusc). O.M= *Oncorhynchus mykiss*. F.h= *Fundulus heteroclitus*. L.m= *Lepomis macrochirus*. G.d=*Gallus domesticus*. M.v=*Mustela vison*.

AP: Acid phosphatase activity. PHL: Phenoloxidase level. NSE: and non-specific esterase activity. ROS: reactive oxygen species production. NO: nitric oxide. NOS: nitric oxide synthetase. MT= Metallothionein. LPO= Lipid peroxidation. CYP 1A1= cytochrome P-450 1A1 isoform. COX-2= cyclooxigenase-2 activity.

The production of reactive oxygen species is among the most common immunotoxicity action mechanisms, and may damage immune system organs through decoupling of electron flow or alterations in antioxidant defenses and the glutathione cycle (Benarjee et al., 2001). Changes in the calcium-dependent mechanisms of lymphoid cells likewise induce modifications in the intracellular levels of this cation in immune system cells (Davila et al., 1995).

Histopathological Strategies

Histopathological exploration of immune system organs is a major tool for identifying immunotoxicant-induced damage (Kuper *et al.*, 2000). This can be done at the coarse level by macroscopic exploration and calculation of the organ/body ratio [I_x %= (lymphatic organ weight / specimen weight)*100], and these measurements should be analyzed by covariance analysis or other statistical tests for nonparametric variables. This is subsequently accompanied by conventional histological evaluations, immunohistodetection, or even electron microscopy determination of damage at the ultra structural level. Organs of choice are the thymus, spleen, lymphatic glands, gastrointestinal associated lymphoid tissue (GALT) or Payer plaques, mucosa associated lymphoid tissue (MALT) and, of course, the bone marrow. However, the choice of an organ will depend on the type of organism studied since structural and anatomical variations exist among different zoological groups. For example, in fish the suprarenal gland performs the same functions as the bone marrow in mammals while, in contrast to these, the thymus is relatively easy to isolate in adult specimens. Infiltration by immune system mononuclear cells forming centers of infection in non lymphoid tissues may also be an indication of immunotoxicity. Description of cell types *in situ*, the relative abundance of these, lymphocyte distribution within the organ, etc. is important. Although these tasks are apparently very extensive, this type of protocol does not require histopathological exploration of all the specimens exposed. The justification of desired probability and predictive power is advisable. A minimum probability of $\alpha = 0.35$ is suggested for immunohistopathological studies. However, some authors consider that the challenge lies in quantitatively relating level of exposure to degree of damage in these tissues (Descotes, 2006). The most commonly used histological techniques are paraffin embedding followed by staining with hematoxylin-eosin. For example, in spleen, description of lymphocyte distribution, B and T-cell germinal centers and periarteriolar lymphocytic aggregations is important. Description of immune activation (relative number of follicles / number of germinal centers) must be considered in lymphatic nodes and Payer plaques. In thymus, description and quantification as far as possible of atrophy, necrosis, apoptosis and other abnormalities such as growth of Hassall's corpuscles is recommended.

Conclusions

Because of the large number of toxic substances, evaluation of their potential risk to immune system function and/or integrity is necessary. Although many studies are available on immunosuppression in both animal models and environmentally exposed humans, there is an evident need for further study of the effects of immunostimulation. At very low concentrations certain toxicants are likely to stimulate function in immune system cells, particularly those that are able to affect the production of certain molecules against infectious-contagious agents and damaged or cancerous cells.

Perspectives

Priority must be given to the synthesis of multiple binding antibodies, recombinant proteins, etc., in order to facilitate immunotoxicological research in most zoological groups, since advance in knowledge will depend on the technical conditions necessary to accomplish this goal.

Acknowledgments

This paper was financed by CONACyT-ICyTDF code 121184 and by IPN, SIP code 20101457. Y. Ortega-Ortega is a graduate DSc student. DSc A. Vega-López, DSc M.L. Domínguez-Lópe, PhD Luis A. Jiménez-Zamudio and PhD Ethel García-Latorre are fellows of Estímulos al Desempeño en Investigación and Comisión y Fomento de Actividades Académicas (Instituto Politécnico Nacional) and Sistema Nacional de Investigadores (SNI, CONACyT, Mexico).

References

Aam BB, Fonnum F. 2006. (+/-)-2-*Chloropropionic acid elevates reactive oxygen species formation in human neutrophil granulocytes*. Toxicology. 228(2-3), 124-134.

Ahmad I, Coelho JP, Mohmood I, Pacheco M, Santos MA, Duarte AC, Pereira E. 2011. *Immunosuppression in the infaunal bivalve Scrobicularia plana environmentally exposed to mercury and association with its accumulation.* Chemosphere. 82(11), 1541-1546.

Anderson SE, Munson AE, Tomblyn S, Meade BJ, Diotte NM. 2008. *The humoral immune response of mice exposed to simulated road paving-like asphalt fumes.* J Immunotoxicol. 5(3), 307-313.

ATSDR, Agency for Toxic Substances and Disease Registry. 2008. *Notice of the Revised Priority List of Hazardous Substances That Will Be the Subject of Toxicological Profiles.* Fed. Reg. 73 (45), 12178-12179

Bálint G, Gergely PJr. 1996. *Clinical immunotoxicity of antirheumatic drugs.* Inflamm. Res. 45(2-Supp), S91-95.

Baken KA, Vandebriel RJ, Pennings JL, Kleinjans JC, van Loveren H. 2007. *Toxicogenomics in the assessment of immunotoxicity*. Methods. 41(1), 132-141.

Baken KA, Pennings JL, Jonker MJ, Schaap MM, de Vries A, van Steeg H, Breit TM, van Loveren H. 2008. *Overlapping gene expression profiles of model compounds provide opportunities for immunotoxicity screening*. Toxicol Appl Pharmacol. 226(1), 46-59.

Black RD, McVey DS, Oehme FW. 1992. *Immunotoxicity in the bovine animal: a review.* Vet. Hum. Toxicol. 34(5), 438-442.

Benarjee, B.D., Seth, V., y Ahmed, R.S. 2001. *Pesticide-induced oxidative stress: perspectives and trends.* Rev. Environ. Health. 16(1), 1-40.

Bernier J, Brousseau P, Krzystyniak K Tryphonas H, Fournier M. 1995. *Immunotoxicy of heavy metals in relation to Great Lakes.* Environ. Health Persp. 103(9), 23-34.

Bondy GS, Pestka JJ. 2000. *Immunomodulation by fungal toxins.* J. Toxicol. Environ. Health B Crit. Rev. 3(2), 109-143.

Boyer IJ. 1989. *Toxicity of dibutylin, tributylin and other organotin compounds to humans and to experimental animals.* Toxicology. 55(3), 253-298.

Blum DJW, Speece RE. 1990. *Determining chemical toxicity to aquatic species. The use of QSARs and surrogate organism.* Environ. Sci. Technol. 24(3), 283-293.

Burastero SE, Paolucci C, Breda D, Ponti J, Munaro B, Sabbioni E. 2006. *Chromium (VI)-induced immunotoxicity and intracellular accumulation in human primary dendritic cells.* Int J Immunopathol Pharmacol. 19(3), 581-591.

Coelho PC, García-Lestón J, Silva SP, da Costa CS, da Costa SC, Coelho MI, Lage BL, Mendez EP, Teixeira JP. 2011. *Geno- and immunotoxic effects on populations living near a mine: a case study of Panasqueira mine in Portugal.* J Toxicol Environ Health A. 74(15-16), 1076-1086.

Cohen MD, Sisco M, Prophete C, Yoshida K, Chen LC, Zelikoff JT, Smee J, Holder AA, Stonehuerner J, Crans DC, Ghio AJ. 2010. *Effects of metal compounds with distinct physicochemical properties on iron homeostasis and antibacterial activity in the lungs: chromium and vanadium.* Inhal Toxicol. 22(2):169-178.

Dansette PM, Bonierbale E, Minoletti C, Beaune PH, Pessayre D, Mansuy D. 1998. *Drug-induced immunotoxicity.* Eur. J. Drug Metab. Pharmacol. 23(4), 443-451.

Das GP, Shaik AP, Jamil K. 2006. *Estimation of apoptosis and necrosis caused by pesticides in vitro on human lymphocytes using DNA diffusion assay.* Drug. Chem. Toxicol. 29, 147-156.

Davila DR, Davis DP, Campbell K, Cambier JC, Zigmond LA, Burchiel SW. 1995. *Role of alterations in Ca(2+)-associated signals pathways in the immunotoxicity of polycyclic aromatic hydrocarbons.* J. Toxicol. Environ. Health. 45(2), 101-126.

Dean JH, Thrumond LM. 1987. *Immunotoxicology: a review.* Toxicol. Pathol. 15(3), 265-271.

De Jong WH, van Loveren H. 2007. *Screening of xenobiotics for direct immunotoxicity in an animal study.* Methods. 4181), 3-8.

Descotes J. 1992. *Immunotoxicology of cadmium.* IARC Sci. Publ. 118, 385-390.

Descotes J. 2006. *Methods of evaluating immunotoxicity.* Expert. Opin. Drug Metab. Toxicol. 2(2), 249-259.

Di Gioacchino, M, Verna N, Di Giampaolo L, Di Claudio F, Turi MC, Perrone A, Petrarca C, Mariani-Constantini R, Sabbioni E, Boscolo P. 2007. *Immunotoxicity and sensitizing capacity of metal compounds depends on speciation.* Int. J. Immunopathol. Pharmacol. 20 (Suppl 2), 15-22.

Duffy-Whritenour JE, Kurtzman RZ, Kennedy S, Zelikoff JT. 2010. *Non-coplanar polychlorinated biphenyl (PCB)-induced immunotoxicity is coincident with alterations in the serotonergic system.* J Immunotoxicol. 7(4), 318-26.

Farahat SA, Rashed LA, Zawilla NH, Farouk SM. 2009. *Effect of occupational exposure to elemental mercury in the amalgam on thymulin hormone production among dental staff.* Toxicol Ind Health. 25(3), 159-167.

Farrer DG, Hueber S, Laiosa MD, Eckles KG, McCabe MJ Jr. 2008. *Reduction of myeloid suppressor cell derived nitric oxide provides a mechanistic basis of lead enhancement of alloreactive CD4(+) T cell proliferation.* Toxicol Appl Pharmacol. 229(2), 135-145.

Fortier M, Omara F, Bernier J, Brousseau P, Fournier M. 2008. *Effects of physiological concentrations of heavy metals both individually and in mixtures on the viability and function of peripheral blood human leukocytes in vitro.* J Toxicol Environ Health A. 71(19), 1327-1337.

Frederick LA, Van Veld PA, Rice CD. 2007. *Bioindicators of immune function in creosote-adapted estuarine killifish, Fundulus heteroclitus.* J Toxicol Environ Health A. 70(17), 1433-1442.

Frisk P, Molin Y, Ilbäck NG. 2008. *Tissue uptake of mercury is changed during the course of a common viral infection in mice.* Environ Res. 106(2), 178-184.

Frouin H, Fortier M, Fournier M. 2010. *Toxic effects of various pollutants in 11B7501 lymphoma B cell line from harbour seal (Phoca vitulina).* Toxicology. 270(2-3), 66-76.

García-Lestón J, Roma-Torres J, Vilares M, Pinto R, Cunha LM, Prista J, Teixeira JP, Mayan O, Pásaro E, Méndez J, Laffon B. 2011. *Biomonitoring of a population of Portuguese workers exposed to lead.* Mutat Res. 721(1), 81-88.

Gardner RM, Nyland JF, Silva IA, Ventura AM, de Souza JM, Silbergeld EK. 2010. *Mercury exposure, serum antinuclear/antinucleolar antibodies, and serum cytokine levels in mining populations in Amazonian Brazil: a cross-sectional study.* Environ Res. 110(4), 345-354.

Gilbert KM, Rowley B, Gomez-Acevedo H, Blossom SJ. 2011. *Coexposure to mercury increases immunotoxicity of trichloroethylene.* Toxicol Sci. 119(2), 281-292.

Gill U, Chu I., Feeley M. 2004. *Polybrominated diphenyl ethers: human tissue levels and toxicology.* Rev. Environ. Contam. Toxicol. 183, 55-97.

Heilmann C, Budtz-Jørgensen E, Nielsen F, Heinzow B, Weihe P, Grandjean P. 2010. *Serum concentrations of antibodies against vaccine toxoids in children exposed perinatally to immunotoxicants.* Environ Health Perspect. 118(10), 1434-1438.

Hermes-Lima, M. 2004. *Oxygen in Biology and Biochemistry: role of free radicals.* In: Storey, K.B. (Ed). Functional Metabolism: Regulation and Adaptation, John Wiley & Sons, Inc. pp 319-368.

Hogan NS, Lee KS, Köllner B, van den Heuvel MR. 2010. *The effects of the alkyl polycyclic aromatic hydrocarbon retene on rainbow trout (Oncorhynchus mykiss) immune response.* Aquat Toxicol. 100(3), 246-254.

Hostýnek JJ. 2002. *Nickel-induced hypersensitivity: etiology, immune reactions, prevention and therapy.* Arch. Dermatol Res. 294(6), 249-267.

Hostýnek JJ. 2006. *Sensitization to nickel: etiology, epidemiology, immune reactions, prevention, and therapy.* Rev. Environ. Health. 21(4), 253-280.

Houben GF, Penninks AH. 1994. *Immunotoxicity of the colour additive caramel III: a review on complicated issues in the safety evaluation of a food additive.* Toxicology. 91(3), 289-302.

Iwanowicz LR, Blazer VS, McCormick SD, Vanveld PA, Ottinger CA. 2009. *Aroclor 1248 exposure leads to immunomodulation, decreased disease resistance and endocrine disruption in the brown bullhead, Ameiurus nebulosus.* Aquat Toxicol. 93(1), 70-82.

Jadhav SH, Sarkar SN, Ram GC, Tripathi HC. 2007. *Immunosuppressive effect of subchronic exposure to a mixture of eight heavy metals, found as groundwater contaminants in different areas of India, through drinking water in male rats.* Arch Environ Contam Toxicol. 53(3), 450-458.

Jusko TA, De Roos AJ, Schwartz SM, Lawrence BP, Palkovicova L, Nemessanyi T, Drobna B, Fabisikova A, Kocan A, Jahnova E, Kavanagh TJ, Trnovec T, Hertz-Picciotto I. 2011. *Maternal and early postnatal polychlorinated biphenyl exposure in relation to total serum immunoglobulin concentrations in 6-month-old infants.* J Immunotoxicol. 8(1), 95-100.

Jörgensen SE. 1990. *Toxicity data and estimation methods.* In: Jörgensen, S.E. (Ed). Modelling in Ecotoxicology. Elsevier, The Netherlands, pp319-332.

Kamlet MJ, Doherty RM, Abbound JL, Abraham MH, Taft RW. 1986. *Linear solvatation energy relationships: 36 Molecular properties solubilities of organic nonelectrolytes in water.* J. Pharm. Sci. 75(4), 338-349.

Khan MI, Islam N, Sahasrabuddhe AA, Mahdi AA, Siddiqui H, Ashquin M, Ahmad I. 2011. *Ubiquitous hazardous metal lead induces TNF-α in human phagocytic THP-1 cells: primary role of ERK 1/2.* J Hazard Mater. 189(1-2), 255-264.

Kier LB. 1981. *Quantitation of solvent polarity based on molecular structure.* J. Pharm. Sci. 70(8), 930-933.

Kuper CF, Harleman JH, Richther-Reichelm HB, Vos JG. 2000. *Histopathologic approaches to detect changes indicative of immunotoxicity.* Toxicol. Pathol. 28(3), 454-466.

Ladics GS. 2007. *Use of SRBC antibody responses for immunotoxicity testing.* Methods. 41(1), 9-19.

Lauriano ER, Calò M, Silvestri G, Zaccone D, Pergolizzi S, Lo Cascio P. 2011. *Mast cells in the intestine and gills of the sea bream, Sparus aurata, exposed to a polychlorinated biphenyl, PCB 126.* Acta Histochem. 2011 May 10. [Epub ahead of print]

Lavoie ET, Wiley F, Grasman KA, Tillitt DE, Sikarskie JG, Bowerman WW. 2007. *Effect of In Ovo exposure to an organochlorine mixture extracted from double crested cormorant eggs (Phalacrocorax auritus) and PCB 126 on immune function of juvenile chickens.* Arch Environ Contam Toxicol. 53(4), 655-661.

Lavoie ET, Grasman KA. 2007. *Effects of in ovo exposure to PCBs 126 and 77 on mortality, deformities and post-hatch immune function in chickens.* J Toxicol Environ Health A. 70(6), 547-558.

Li Q, Nagahara N, Takahashi H, Takeda K, Okumura K, Minami, M. 2002. *Organophosphorus pesticides markedly inhibit the activities of natural killer, cytotoxic T lymphocyte and lymphokine-activated killer: a proposed inhibiting mechanism via granzyme inhibition.* Toxicology 172, 181-190.

Li Q, Nakadai A, Ishizaki M, Morimoto K, Ueda A, Krensky AM, Kawada T. 2005. *Dimethyl 2,2-dichlorovinyl phosphate (DDVP) markedly decreases the expression of perforin, granzyne A and granulysin in human NK-92CI cell line.* Toxicology. 213, 107-116.

Li Q, Kawada T. 2006. *The mechanism of organophosphorus pesticides-induced inhibition of cytolytic activity of killer cells.* Cell. Mol. Immunol. 3, 171-178.

Liu J, Qu W, Kadiiska MB. 2009. *Role of oxidative stress in cadmium toxicity and carcinogenesis.* Toxicol Appl Pharmacol. 238(3), 209-214.

Luebke RW, Chen DH, Diertert R, Yang Y, Kin M, Luster MI, *et al.* 2006. *The comparative immunotoxicity of five selected compounds following development of adult exposure.* J Toxicol. Environ. Health B Crit. Rev. 9(1), 1-26.

Lugo RS, Nathalí G, Villalobos de B LB, Mairin L. 2006. *Immunological response of the freshwater fish Colossoma macropomum as a biomarker of copper exposure.* Bull Environ Contam Toxicol. 77(6), 925-930.

Luster MI, Rosenthal GJ. 1993. *Chemical agents and the immune response. Environ.* Health Perspect. 100, 219-226.

Martin PA, Mayne GJ, Bursian FS, Tomy G, Palace V, Pekarik C, Smits J. 2007. Immunotoxicity of the commercial polybrominated diphenyl ether mixture DE-71 in ranch mink (*Mustela vison*). Environ Toxicol Chem. 26(5), 988-997.

Merk HF, Sachs B, Baron J. 2001. The skin: target organ in Immunotoxicology of small-molecular-weight compounds. Skin Pharmacol. Appl. Skin Physiol. 14(6), 419-430.

Messiha FS. 1994. *Developmental toxicity of cesium in the mouse.* Gen Pharmacol. 25(3), 395-400.

Mishra PK, Panwar H, Bhargava A, Gorantla VR, Jain SK, Banerjee S, Maudar KK. 2008. *Isocyanates induces DNA damage, apoptosis, oxidative stress, and inflammation in cultured human lymphocytes.* J Biochem Mol Toxicol. 22(6), 429-440.

Mottin E, Caplat C, Mahaut ML, Costil K, Barillier D, Lebel JM, Serpentini A. 2010. *Effect of in vitro exposure to zinc on immunological parameters of haemocytes from the marine gastropod Haliotis tuberculata.* Fish Shellfish Immunol. 29(5), 846-853.

Moszczyński P. 1999. *Immunological disorders in men exposed to metallic mercury vapour: a review.* Cent., Eur. J. Public Health. 7(1), 10-14.

Murray MJ, Kerkvliet NI, Ward EC, Dean JH. 1985. *Models for the evaluation of tumor resistance following chemical or drug exposure.* In: Immunotoxicology and immunopharmacology. Dean, J.H., Luster, M.I., Munson, A.E., Amos, H. (Eds) Raven Press, New York. pp 113-122.

Nad P, Pistl J, Skalická M, Koréneková B, Demeterová M, Bindas L, Mal'a P. 2009. *Effect of oral cadmium and zinc application on leukocytes biological activity in Japanese quails (Coturnix coturnix japonica).* Berl Munch Tierarztl Wochenschr. 122(9-10), 364-369.

Nain S, Smits JE. 2011. *Subchronic lead exposure, immunotoxicology and increased disease resistance in Japanese quail (Corturnix coturnix japonica).* Ecotoxicol Environ Saf. 74(4), 787-792.

Nakayama A, Riesen I, Köllner B, Eppler E, Segner H. 2008. *Surface marker-defined head kidney granulocytes and B lymphocytes of rainbow trout express benzo[a]pyrene-inducible cytochrome P4501A protein.* Toxicol Sci. 103(1), 86-96.

Pallardy M, Biola A, Lebrec H, Bréard J. 1999. *Assessment of apoptosis in xenobiotic-induced immunotoxicity.* Methods. 19(1), 36-47.

Pathak N, Khandelwal S. 2008. *Impact of cadmium in T lymphocyte subsets and cytokine expression: differential regulation by oxidative stress and apoptosis.* Biometals. 21(2), 179-187.

Peakall DB, Shugart LR.1994. *Biomarkers. In: Mayers, R.A. (Ed). Environmental Analysis and Remediation.* JohnWiley & Sons, New York. pp 732-755.

Pieters R, Albers R. 1999. *Screening test for autoimmune-related immunotoxicity. Environ.* Health Prespect. 107(5-Supp), 673-677.

Pruett SB, Ensley DK, Crittenden PL. 1993. *The role of chemical-induced stress response in immunosupression: a review of quantitative associations and cause-effect relationships between chemical-induced stress responses and immunosuppression.* J. Toxicol. Environ. Health. 39(2), 163-192.

Repetto M. 1997. *Tránsito de los xenobióticos en el organismo. Toxicocinética.* In: Repetto, M. (Ed). Toxicología Fundamental, Díaz de Santos, Madrid, pp.47-82.

Reynaud S, Deschaux P. 2006. *The effects of polyaromatic hydrocarbons on the immune system of fish: A review.* Aquat. Toxicol. 77, 229-238.

Rosato E, Giovannetti A, Rossi C, Menghi G, Pisarri S, Salsano F. 2009. *Recurrent infections in patients with nickel allergic hypersensitivity.* J Biol Regul Homeost Agents. 23(3), 173-180.

Ross P, de Swart R, Addison R, van Loveren H, Vos J, Osterhaus A. 1996. *Contaminant-induced immunotoxicity in harbor seals: wildlife at risk?* Toxicology. 11282), 157-169.

Safe S, Mason G, Sawyer T, Zacharewski T, Harris M, Yao C, Keys B, Farrell K, Holcomb M, Davis D, *et al.* 1989. *Development and validation of in vitro induction assays for toxic halogenated aromatic mixtures: a review.* Toxicol. Ind. Health. 5(5), 757-775.

Schellenberger MT, Grova N, Willième S, Farinelle S, Prodhomme EJ, Muller CP. 2009. *Modulation of benzo[a]pyrene induced immunotoxicity in mice actively immunized with a B[a]P-diphtheria toxoid conjugate.* Toxicol Appl Pharmacol. 240(1), 37-45.

Sparfel L, Pinel-Marie ML, Boize M, Koscielny S, Desmots S, Pery A, Fardel O. 2010. *Transcriptional signature of human macrophages exposed to the environmental contaminant benzo(a)pyrene.* Toxicol Sci. 114(2), 247-259.

Selgrade MK. 2007. Immunotoxicity: the risk is real. Toxicol. Sci. 100(2), 328-332.

Silbergeld, E.K., Silva, I.A., y Nyland, J.F. 2005. *Mercury and autoimmunity: implicantins for occupational and environmental health.* Toxicol Appl. Pharmacol. 207(2 Supp), 282-292.

Sim E. 1989. *Drug-induced immune-complex disease.* Complement Inflamm. 6(2), 119-126.

Sørmo EG, Larsen HJ, Johansen GM, Skaare JU, Jenssen BM. 2009. *Immunotoxicity of polychlorinated biphenyls (PCB) in free-ranging gray seal pups with special emphasis on dioxin-like congeners.* J Toxicol Environ Health A. 72(3-4), 266-276.

Trickler WJ, Lantz SM, Murdock RC, Schrand AM, Robinson BL, Newport GD, Schlager JJ, Oldenburg SJ, Paule MG, Slikker W Jr, Hussain SM, Ali SF. 2010. *Silver nanoparticle induced blood-brain barrier inflammation and increased permeability in primary rat brain microvessel endothelial cells.* Toxicol Sci. 118(1), 160-170.

Tryphonas H. 1995. *Immunotoxicity of PCBs (Aroclors) in relation to Great Lakes.* Environ. Health Perspect. 103 (9-Supp), 35-46.

U.S.DHHS, U.S. Department of Health and Human Services. 1997. *Registry of the toxic effects of chemical substances (RTECS) comprehensive guide to the RTECS. Sweet* D. V. (Ed.) National Institute for Occupational Safety and Health, Cincinnati, Ohio. U.S.A. 80 p.

van der Oost R, Beyer J, Vermeulen NPE. 2003. *Fish bioaccumulation and biomarkers in environmental risk assessment: a review.* Environ. Toxicol. Pharmacol. 13, 57-149.

van Loveren H, Ross PS, Osterhaus AD, Vos JG. 2000. *Contaminant-induced immunosuppression and mass mortalities among harbor seals*. Toxicol. Lett. 112-113, 319-324.

Vega-López A, Galar-Martínez M, Jiménez-Orozco FA, García-Latorre E, Domínguez-López ML. 2007. *Gender related differences in the oxidative stress response to PCB exposure in an endangered goodeid fish (Girardinichthys viviparus)*. Comp. Biochem. Physiol. Part A. 146, 672-678.

Vega-López A, Jiménez-Orozco FA, García-Latorre E, Domínguez-López ML. 2008a. *Estrogenic effects of polychlorinated biphenyls and relation to cytochrome P4501A activity in the endangered goodeid fish Ameca splendens.* Environ. Toxicol. Chem. 27(4), 963-969.

Vega-López A, Jiménez-Orozco FA, García-Latorre E, Domínguez-López ML. 2008b. *Oxidative stress response in an endangered goodeid fish (Girardinichthys viviparus) by exposure to water from its extant localities.* Ecotoxicol. Environ. Saf. 71, 94-103.

Vega-López A, Jiménez-Orozco FA, Jiménez-Zamudio LA, García-Latorre E, Domínguez-López ML. 2009. *Phase I enzyme induction in Girardinichthys viviparus, an endangered goodeid fish, exposed to water from its native localities enriched with polychlorinated biphenyls*. Arch. Environ. Contam. Toxicol. 57, 561–570

Vijayavel K, Gopalakrishnan S, Thiagarajan R, Thilagam H. 2009. *Immunotoxic effects of nickel in the mud crab Scylla serrata.* Fish Shellfish Immunol. 26(1), 133-139.

Vos JG, van Loveren H. 1998. *Experimental studies on immunosuppression: how do they predict for man?* Toxicology. 129(1), 13-26.

WHO, *United Nations Environment Programme International Labor Office. 1986: In Inmunotoxicology: Development of predictive test for determining the immunotoxic potential of chemical*. Report of a Technical Review Meeting. WHO Press, London.

WHO, International Programme on Chemistry Safety (IPCS). 1993. *Biomarkers and risk assessment: concepts and principles*. Environmental Health Criteria 155. WHO, Geneva.

Whyte JJ, Jueng RE, Schmitt CJ, Tillitt DE. 2000. *Ethoxiresorufin o-deethylase (EROD) activity in fish a biomarker of chemical exposure*. In: McClellan R.O (Ed). Crit. Rev. Toxicol. 30, 347-570.

Wu RSS, Siu WHL, Shin PKS. 2005. *Induction, adaptation and recovery of biological responses: Implications for environmental monitoring*. Mar. Poll. Bull. 51, 623-634.

Zelikoff JT, Raymond A, Carlson E, Beaman JR, Anderson M. 2000. *Biomarkers of Immunotoxicology in fish: from the lab to the ocean*. Toxicol. Lett. 112-113, 325-331.

Zinedine A, Soriano JM, Olto JC, Mañes J. 2007. *Review on the toxicity, occurrence, metabolisms, detoxification, regulations and intake of zearalenone: An oestrogenic mycotoxin.* Food Chem. Toxicol. 45, 1-18.

In: Xenobiotics: New Research
Editors: Saul F. Castaneda and Mauro L. Emerson
ISBN: 978-1-61942-616-0

Chapter 2

POTENTIAL OF WEAK CYP1A INDUCERS FOR THE PREVENTION AND THERAPIES OF CHEMICALLY-INDUCED CANCER

Maria Perepechaeva[1]*, Yulia Sidorova[1,2] and Alevtina Grishanova[1]

[1]Institute of Molecular Biology and Biophysics SB RAMS, Timakova Str. 2, Novosibirsk, Russia

[2]Institute of Biotechology, Viikki Biocenter, Viikinkaari 9, PL 56, 00014 - University of Helsinki, Helsinki, Finland

ABSTRACT

Cytochromes P450 1A sub-family (CYP1A1 and CYP1A2) are well-known metabolizers of anthropogenic compounds such as polycyclic aromatic hydrocarbons (PAHs) and arylamines. They catalyze all metabolic reactions occurring with PAHs in the organism including the ones resulting in the formation of carcinogenic, mutagenic and teratogenic substances. PAH in their intact, exogenous form usually do not produce adverse effects on the organism (except rare cases of acute poisoning with extremely high doses), however, their metabolites are able to bind and damage macromolecules in the cells. PAHs characterized by specific physical and chemical properties: they are hydrophobic, planar molecules with the size of approximately 6.8 x 13.7 Å. In organisms, PAH activate expression of CYP1A and serve as their substrates. PAH-like inducers of CYP1A are called "classic" inducers. They increase CYP1A activity hundreds fold, undergo metabolic activation and, afterwards, become able to promote the development of dangerous diseases including chemically-induced cancer.

Recent studies demonstrate an increasing number of non-PAH-like CYP1A inducers, which have different physical and chemical properties. These substances include endogenous compounds and food components, such as indoles, flavonoids, vitamins, and some others. They are so-called "weak" or "non-classical" CYP1A inducers and they increase the enzyme activity not more than several times. This mild activation of CYP1A

* Correspondent author E-mail: perepech@soramn.ru. Tel/Fax: +7 (383) 335-9847.

by naturally-occuring substances probably has a physiological function and is not dangerous for organisms.

At least some “weak” CYP1A inducers are able to inhibit the effect of "classic" inducers such as 2,3,7,8-Tetrachlorodibenzodioxin (TCDD) or benzo(a)pyrene in the case of combined administration. Since classic inducers are metabolized by CYP1A to reactive intermediates able to cause chemically-induced cancer and other diseases, the suppression of CYP1A activity might be a useful tool for their prevention and/or management. Thus, detailed understanding of molecular mechanisms underlying this phenomenon is required. Further investigation of “weak” CYP1A inducers might result in the development of new medical strategies to prevent or fight adverse effects of PAH-like anthropogenic xenobiotics.

ABBREVIATIONS

3-MC, 3-methylcholanthrene; ADPF, AhR degradation promoting factor; AhR, aryl hydrocarbon receptor; AINT, Arnt interacting protein; AhRR, aryl hydrocarbon receptor repressor; Arnt, Ah receptor nuclear translocator; BP, benzo(α)pyrene; C/EBPβ, CCAA/enhancer binding protein β, CYP1A1, cytochrome P450 1A1; CYP1A2, cytochrome P450 1A2; Hif1α, hypoxia-inducible transcription factor α, HO-1, heme oxygenase 1; Hsp90, heat shock protein 90; NRE, negative regulatory element; PAHs, polycyclic aromatic hydrocarbons; ROS, reactive oxygen species; TCDD, 2,3,7,8-Tetrachlorodibenzodioxin; XAP2, hepatitis B virus X-associated protein 2;XRE, xenobiotic responsive element.

INTRODUCTION

Living organisms continuously interact with many chemical compounds in the environment which are not integrated in the biochemical reactions. These chemicals are named xenobiotics, some of them have natural origin (alkaloids, metabolites of plants, toxins), the others are anthropogenic (drugs, industrial chemicals, pesticides and others). A microsomal monooxygenase system (the system of biotransformation of xenobiotics) enzymatically converts hydrophobic exogeneous substances to more hydrophilic molecules that can be excreted from the organisms by kidneys and intestine (with urine and bile). Metabolism of xenobiotics usually occurs in two phases: the modification and conjugation. Reactions of the first phase are carried out by a super-family of hemoproteins, called cytochromes P450 (CYPs), they catalyze oxygenation of the substrates which results in the formation of more polar and reactive molecules. Subsequently, enzymes of the 2nd phase (glutathione-S-transferases, UDP-glucuronosyl transferases, quinone reductases, N-acetyltransferases, methyltransferases) promote the formation of conjugates that are water soluble, even more polar and, as a rule, less toxic. Thus, enzymes of the second phase of xenobiotic metabolism are very important for the excretion of exogeneous substances, however, in current review, we will focus only on enzymes of the first phase, in particular on cytochromes P450 of 1A sub-family.

Cytochrome P450 was discovered as a gemoprotein that absorbs light at 450 nm wavelength. For many years it was thought that this enzyme did not have strict substrate specificity because of its ability to metabolize a wide range of different chemical substances.

However, the existence of multiple isoforms of cytochrome P450 was demonstrated. Isoforms differ in molecular weight, amino acid sequence and substrate specificity. On the basis of similarity of amino acid sequences, they are organized into sub-families, families and altogether constitute the super-family of cytochromes P450.

CYP1A sub-family of cytochromes P450 in mammals consists of two members: CYP1A1 and CYP1A2. These enzymes metabolize the most common classes of carcinogens - polycyclic aromatic hydrocarbons (PAHs), such as benzo(α)pyrene (BP), 3-methylcholanthrene (3-MC) (The structures of these compounds are presented in Figure. 1) and halogenated aromatic hydrocarbons such as dioxin and related compounds. CYP1A play an important part in the bioactivation of these chemicals, catalyzing production of their epoxides and other compounds that are highly reactive and are able to bind to cell components (Whitlock, 1999; Ma, 2001) exerting mutagenic, toxic and carcinogenic effects. Thus, CYP1A are extensively studied in the context of chemically-induced carcinogenesis.

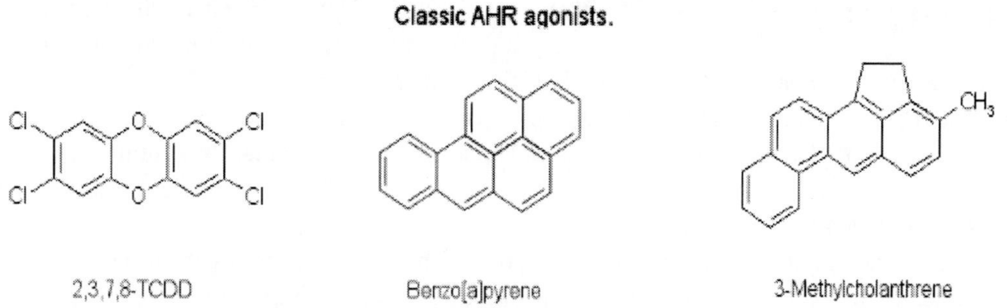

Figure 1. Examples of chemical structure of "classic" AhR ligands.

An important property of xenobiotic-biotransforming enzymes in general and CYP1A sub-family in particular is their capability for induction. Usually, this induction is favorable because it promotes effective elimination of resulting lipophilic compounds and prevents their accumulation in the cells (Whitlock, 1999; Ma, 2001). However, in some cases, induction may have adverse consequences because of the formation of reactive intermediates able to damage cellular macromolecules. PAHs and related chemicals stimulate activity of CYP1A hundreds fold and they are called "classic" inducers of these enzymes. However, in this case, the induction has rather negative consequences, because of the bioactivation of PAHs by CYP1A.

Induction of CYP1A is mediated by aryl hydrocarbon receptor (AhR) which is a ligand-activated protein belonging to the super-family of nuclear receptors. In an inactive state, AhR is located in the cytoplasm in a complex with other proteins that support it in the conformation facilitating ligand binding. After binding to the ligand, AhR dissociates from its cytosolic partners, moves to the nucleus and dimerizes with Arnt (Ah receptor nuclear translocator). Subsequently, AhR/Arnt heterodimer binds to xenobiotic responsive elements (XREs) in the CYP1A1/2 gene enhancer and this finally leads to the initiation of CYP1A1/2 transcription (Ma, 2001).

The problem of mass appearances of diseases associated with intoxication by chlorinated aromatic compounds and dioxin-like compounds - AhR ligands and inducers of CYP1A emerged in the first half of 20th century due to the massive development of the chemical industry. The number of dioxin-related accidents has already been reported and there are no guarantees that similar cases won't happen in the future. In addition, PAHs are contained in the emissions from thermal power generators, present in exhaust gases of internal combustion engines and in tobacco smoke. The main source of BP in the cities is car exhaust. Environmental control measures can be pursued to reduce the amount of harmful emissions, but their complete elimination is not real. In addition, no dose of PAH is really harmless (due to their lipofilicity these compounds might accumulate in the organism up to the toxic concentration).

Acute intoxication by dioxins causes a chloracne (a chronic skin disease), porphyria, transient hepatotoxicity, neurotoxicity. Long-term exposure leads to neural system damage, endocrine and immune system damage, atherosclerosis, hypertension, diabetes and vascular ocular changes (Pelclová et al., 2006; Céspedes et al., 2010; Marinković et al., 2010). Dioxins exert teratogenic, autoimmunic and carcinogenic effects such as gastrointestinal neoplasms and lymphohemopoietic neoplasms formation, lung cancer and breast cancer development and others (Céspedes et al., 2010; Marinković et al., 2010). In experimental animals, exposure to TCDD results in hepatic damage, thymic atrophy, immune dysfunction and cancer development (Birnbaum, 1994). It should be mentioned that CYP1A is expressed predominantly in the lungs of humans, whereas rodents have mainly liver localization of CYP1A. Thus, PAHs are expected to exert adverse effects predominantly in human lungs. It is supported by the fact that some polymorphic variants of CYP1A1 are associated with lung cancer (Smith et al., 2001).

Current treatment efforts for conditions caused by PAHs are focused on combating the consequences of exposure to these pollutants but do not deal with the cause of these disorders on a molecular level. According to the general belief, most, if not all, adverse effects of PAHs are mediated via the induction of an AhR-dependent signaling pathway which results in the bioactivation of these chemicals. That is why it is important to continue to investigate the mechanisms of "classic" AhR ligands action and search for the novel ways to reduce the dangerous effects of PAHs

Over the past two decades, the number of compounds activating AhR and its targets but being structurally different from PAHs has been reported. Among these compounds are molecules of natural origin such as indoles, flavonoids, vitamins, physiological metabolic products (Denison and Nagy, 2003; Nguyen and Bradfield; 2008).They activate AhR targets to a much lower extent than PAHs (not more than several times) (Denison and Nagy, 2003) and that's why they are called "weak" or "non-classic" inducers. Interestingly, these naturally-occuring molecules can interfere with CYP1A induction produced by PAHs and thus, they might provide new alternatives to prevent and/or treat adverse consequences of exposure to these environmental pollutants. In this paper, we made an attempt to describe the spectrum of "weak" CYP1A inducers, their ability to neutralize the effects of PAHs on AhR targets and potential molecular mechanisms underlying this phenomenon.

AHR STRUCTURE, FUNCTION AND SIGNALING. MECHANISM OF CYP1A INDUCTION

Enzyme induction might occur on different levels: by an activation of transcription of correspondent gene, by mRNA stabilization and by translational or post-translational modifications of synthesized protein. Cytochrome P450 isoforms might be induced by all mechanisms described above. However, CYP1A1 was shown to be activated exclusively on a transcriptional level through an AhR-dependent signal transduction pathway (Ma, 2001). In contrast, CYP1A2 activation can occur on both transcriptional level, through the AhR-dependent or AhR-independent signaling pathway and post-transcriptional level (Quattrochi et al., 1994; Raffalli-Mathieu et al., 1997).

AhR is a ligand-activated transcription factor belonging to the super-family of nuclear receptors. It is a member of the basic helix-loop-helix/Per-Arnt-Sim (bHLH/PAS) transcription factor family which includes a circadian oscillator protein Per, AhR nuclear translocator (Arnt), neurodevelopmental factors Sim and hypoxia-inducible transcription factors Hif1α (Minsavage et al., 2004). AhR belongs to the so-called "orphan" receptors for which endogenous ligands and activators had not been identified for a long time or remain unknown (Beischlag et al., 2008). AhR contains several domains with different functions: bHLH domain, PAS domain, three transactivation domains (Ma, 2001; Ramadoss and Perdew, 2005) and inhibitory domain (Figure 2). bHLH domain encompass the basic region responsible for the binding to DNA. PAS domain includes two regions: PAS A which mediates AhR/Arnt dimerization and PAS B which contains a ligand-binding site.

There are also evidences that the PAS B part of AhR might exert an inhibitory effect on AhR transformation to DNA binding form (Soshilov and Denison, 2008). The transactivation domains mediate the transfer of the signal from the enhancer to the promoter but it is not clear which factors and co-factors participate in this process (Whitlock, 1999; Ma, 2001). An inhibitory domain blocks the transactivating functions of AhR and Arnt (Ma et al., 1995; Whitlock, 1999; Soshilov and Denison, 2008).

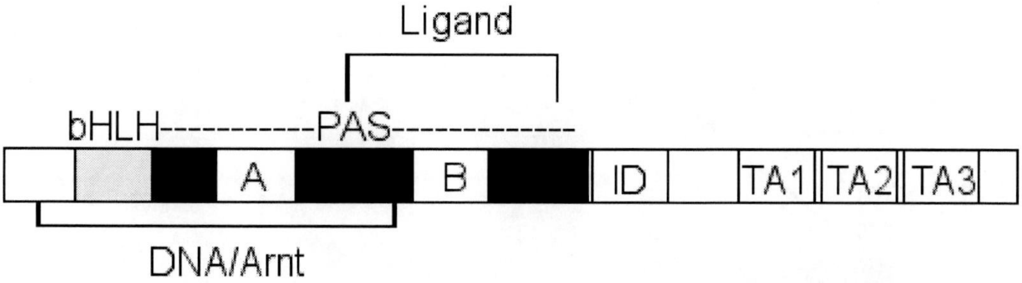

Figure 2. The structure of aryl hydrocarbon receptor (AhR). bHLH- basic-helix-loop-helix domain; PAS- Per-Arnt-Sim domain, A- region A of PAS domain; B – region B of PAS domain; ID - inhibitory domain; TA1-3 - transactivation domains 1-3; DNA/Arnt - region responsible for the binding to DNA and mediating AhR/Arnt dimerization; ligand – refers to the part of the protein responsible for the ligand binding.

When inactive, AhR is located in the cytoplasm in complex with its associated proteins which are two molecules of heat shock protein 90 (Hsp90), c-Src tyrosine kinase, the hepatitis

B virus X-associated protein 2 (XAP2) and the co-chaperone p23 (Enan and Matsumura, 1996; Kazlauskas et al., 2000). Hsp90 functions as a chaperone. It maintains the AhR in the conformation that is unable to bind DNA, but favorable for the binding of the ligand (Carver et al., 1994; Beischlag et al., 2008). p23 co-chaperone stabilizes AhR-Hsp90 interaction and mediates ligand-induced (Petrulis and Perdew, 2002) release of Hsp90 from the Ah-receptor complex after ligand binding (Kazlauskas et al., 2000; Harper et al., 2006). XAP2 protects the ligand-free form of AhR from ubiquitination and degradation and furthermore, the association of XAP2 with AhR is determined by the functional Hsp90 state as well as p23 (Kazlauskas et al., 2000).

Upon ligand binding, the cytosolic complex described above dissociates and AhR in complex with ligand moves to the nuclei where it dimerizes with Arnt. The AhR/Arnt heterodimer then binds to XREs in the *CYP1A1/2* gene enhancer; this stimulates recruitment of basic transcription factors to the promoter of these genes and finally leads to the initiation of their transcription (Ma, 2001). The scheme of an AhR-dependent signal transduction pathway is presented in Figure 3.

It is known that protein kinases are involved in the regulation of nuclear receptors-mediated signaling. An AhR-dependent signal transduction pathway is associated and regulated by the processes of phosphorylation. Both AhR and Arnt are phosphoproteins. AhR is phosphorylated on threonine residues (Delescluse et al., 2000), whereas human Arnt is phosphorylated on serine, threonine and tyrosine residues (Levine and Perdew, 2001). Arnt phosphorylation is required for dimerization with AhR, while AhR phosphorylation is required for the binding of the AhR/Arnt complex to DNA (Ma, 2001). It was shown that the transactivation potential of human Arnt can be modulated by both protein kinase C and protein kinase A (Long et al., 1999). It is in accordance with a previous observation of Machemer and Tukey, who demonstrated that protein kinase C was involved in the regulation of TCDD-induced CYP1A1 expression *in vitro* using a luciferase gene under the control of the human CYP1A1 promoter (Machemer and Tukey, 2005).

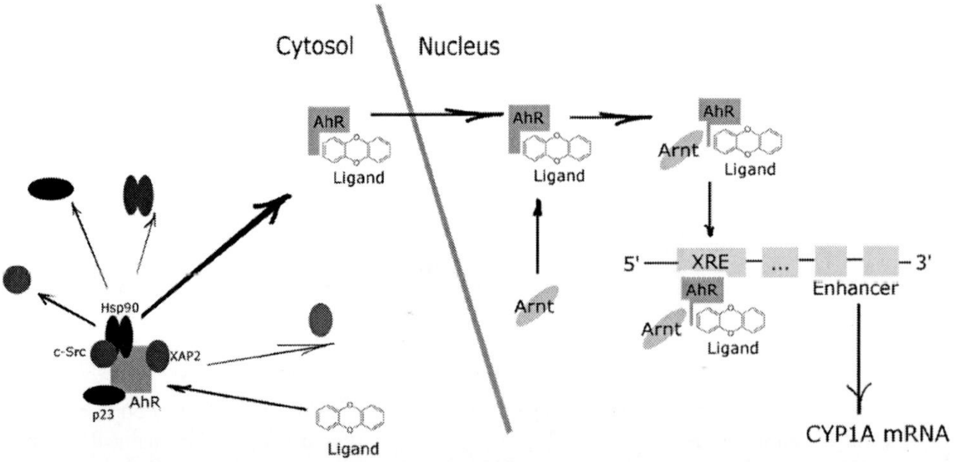

Figure 3. The scheme of the AhR-dependent signal transduction. Before ligand binding, AhR locates in cytoplasm in complex with other proteins (Hsp90, XAP2, p23, c-Src). Ligand binding leads to translocation of AhR to nuclei where it forms a dimer with Arnt. AhR/Arnt dimer binds enhancer of target gene which results in theirs expression.

In addition to its function as a xenobiotics' receptor, AhR plays an important role in several physiological processes, such as immune response, female reproductive functions, cell cycle progression, in normal vascular and liver development (Hernández-Ochoa et al., 2009; Ma et al., 2009; Fujii-Kuriyama and Kawajiri, 2010). Mice lacking AhR have vascular abnormalities in the eyes and kidneys, portal vascular hypertrophy, depletion of splenic lymphocytes, skin lesions, pyloric hyperplasia of the gastrointestinal tract, cardiomegaly, hypertension, hepatic aberrations and impaired reproductive function. In addition, survival of AhR knock-out pups was impaired (40–50% of them died neonatally). This is most likely attributed to the multiple developmental defects in the cardiovascular and immune systems of mice lacking AhR (Harstad et al., 2006; Nguyen and Bradfield; 2008). Full knock-outs of Arnt die before embryonic day 10. However, Arnt interact with other proteins like hypoxia-inducible transcription factor α (Hif1α) and is involved in other signaling pathways such as the ones controlling response to hormones (for example, to estrogens). Thus, a severe phenotype of animals lacking Arnt most likely is not related to its function in xenobiotic metabolism. It might rather be attruibuted to an abnormal response to hypoxia or severe defects in the endocrine system (Gunton et al., 2005; Rüegg et al., 2008).

Involvement of AhR in normal physiological processes and development implies the existence of naturally-occuring and/or endogenous ligands of this receptor. During the past 2 decades the number of non-anthropogenic molecules structurally different from PAHs that activate AhR-dependent targets has been identified. They are overviewed in the following chapter.

Overview of Weak CYP1A Inducers

Identified groups of non-PAH-like compounds weakly activating CYP1A1 are described below. Part of them was demonstrated to serve as AhR ligands, for others the mode of action remains unknown. These molecules activate CYP1A at least 5 times less efficient than PAHs or other classic inducers and that's why they are called weak CYP1A inducers (Astorg et al., 1997; Allen et al., 2001; Sidorova et al., 2004; Sidorova et al., 2005).

Indole-Containing Chemicals

The substances of natural origin such as a component of cruciferous vegetables indole-3-carbinol, ultraviolet photoproducts and some metabolites of tryptophan: tryptamine (Figure 4) and indole acetic acid as well as plant-derived compounds indirubin (used as a drug against leukemia in Chineese medicine) and indigo dye are weak aryl hydrocarbon receptor ligands (Heath-Pagliuso et al., 1998; Adachi et al., 2001; Helferich and Denison, 1991; Nguyen and Bradfield, 2008). Some derivatives of fungi-produced antibiotic tryptanthrin such as 8-methyltryptanthrin, 8-chlorotryptanthrin, and 8-bromotryptanthrin induced CYP1A1 mRNA and protein in primary culture of rat hepatocytes and in Hepa-1 mouse hepatoma cells. It was also demonstrated that these compounds might stimulate the transfer of AhR to nuclei but their direct binding to AhR was not studied (Schrenk et al., 1999; Schrenk et al., 1999).

Arachidonic Acid Metabolites

It is known that several prostaglandins (for example, prostaglandin G2 (Figure 4) (Denison and Nagy, 2003) activate the AhR signaling pathway and downstream targets including CYP1A1 in mouse hepatoma cells in culture. In addition, they have some affinity to AhR and might displace radioactively-labeled TCDD from this receptor (Seidel et al., 2001).

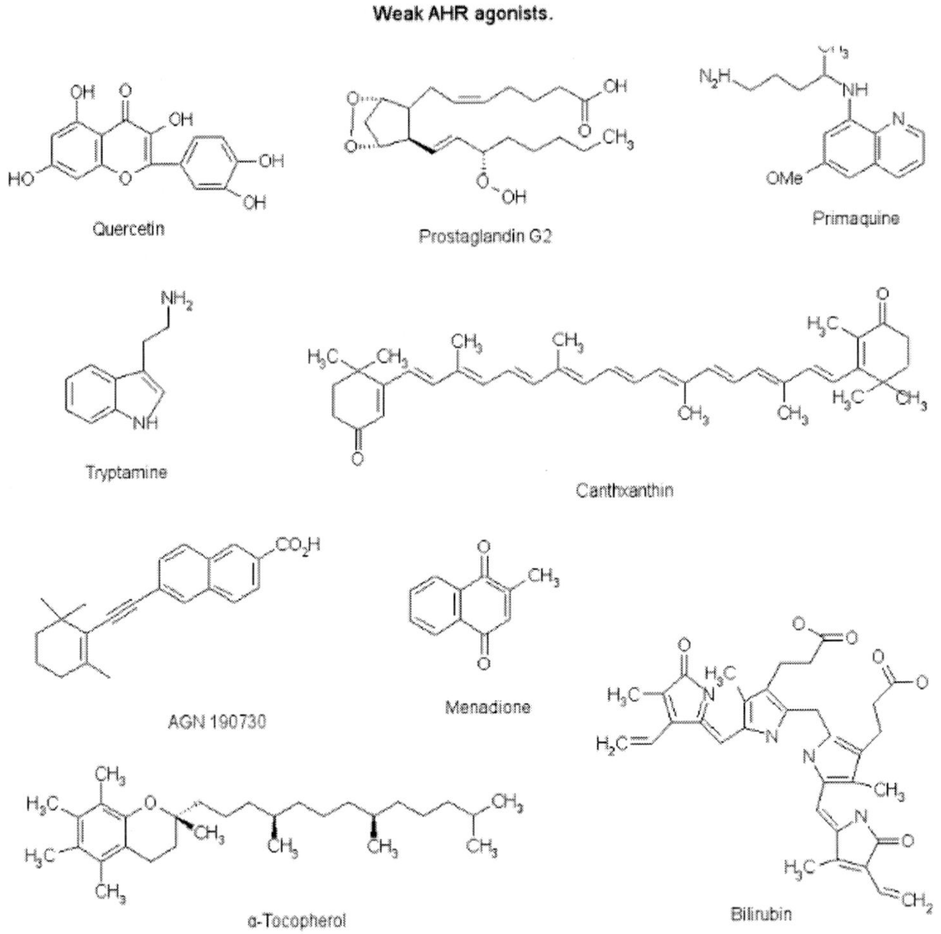

Figure 4. Examples of the chemical structure of "weak" AhR ligands.

Heme Metabolites

Bilirubin (Figure 4) and biliverdin, released by pathological hemolysis can activate CYP1A1/2 through the Ah-receptor signal transduction pathway and serve as AhR ligands (Phelan et al., 1998). These metabolites are potential candidate molecules mediating ultra-sound-induced activation of CYP1A in the rat liver (Grishanova, Zueva, 2000).

Polyphenols and Flavonoids

Several flavonoids including 6,2',4'-trimethoxyflavone and dietary flavonols quercetin (Figure 4) (found in fruits and vegetables) and kaempferol (found in many plant sources) were identified recently as AhR ligands (Ciolino et al., 1999; Murray et al., 2010). The last 2 molecules were also able to displace [^{3}H]TCDD from the cytosolic AhR (Ciolino et al., 1999). Curcumin, a yellow pigment of *Curcuma longa,* activated DNA-binding capacity of the AhR, stimulated a rapid accumulation of *CYP1A1* mRNA and increased CYP1A1 activity in cultured cells. This polyphenol was also able to compete with TCDD for binding to AhR. Authors suggest that curcumin might be a natural ligand and substrate of the AhR pathway (Garg et al., 2008; Ciolino et al., 1998).

VITAMINS

Carotinoids

Canthxanthin (Figure 4), astaxanthin and apo-80-carotinal are able to induce CYP1A1 activity in rats and mice (Denison and Nagy, 2003). Synthetic retinoids: AGN 190730 (Figure 4) and AGN 192837, were found to stimulate CYP1A1 transcription via AhR-dependent pathway in Hepa-1c1c7 cells (Gambone er al., 2002). For these molecules, direct binding to AhR or competition with TCDD was not demonstrated. Suggested mechanism of their action is associated with interactions between AhR-dependent signal transduction and the retinoic acid-signaling pathway (Murphy et al., 2007).

α-Tocopherol (Vitamin E)

We previously demonstrated that nutritional vitamin α-tocopherol (Figure 4) induced CYP1A in rat liver. The ability of this substance to bind to AhR was not studied. However, the induction of CYP1A1 occurred on transcriptional level which might indicate the involvement of AhR-dependent pathway of signal transduction. CYP1A2 was activated by vitamin E on the post-transcriptional level (Sidorova et al., 2004).

Menadione (Vitamin K3)

We also identified menadione (Figure 3) - a synthetic analogue of vitamin K as a weak transcriptional inducer of CYP1A (Sidorova et al., 2005). According to our unpublsihed data (Sidorova et al., unpublished), menadione stimulated AhR/Arnt binding to XRE, although it is not clear whether it is an AhR ligand.

Other known weak inducers of AhR-dependent signaling transduction are an insecticide *carbaryl,*; an anti-malarial agent primaquine (Figure 4) (Bohonowych and Denison, 2007), and benzimidazole drugs such as omeprazole and thiabendazole (Lemaire et al., 2004). The last two molecules were demonstrated to be weak AhR ligands.

To summarize, weak inducers might activate AhR-dependent targets, in particularly, CYP1A by various mechanisms. First of all, AhR might bind structurally diverse compounds. This promiscuity might be explained by the structure of its ligand-binding pocket. Low-affinity and high-affinity AhR ligands were demonstrated to interact with different amino acid residues of an AhR ligand-binding pocket and this might result in the interacting with the active center of the AhR with different affinities (Backlund and Ingelman-Sundberg, 2004). Secondly, compounds activating CYPs do not necessary interact with AhR in their native unmodified form. It is possible that their metabolites have affinity to AhR (Delescluse et al., 2000). Finally, these molecules can activate another signaling pathway(s) which has cross-talks with an AhR-dependent signal transduction pathway and thus, stimulate the last one indirectly.

Mechanisms of Inhibition of AhR Activation and CYP1A Induction

The level of constitutive expression of CYP1A1 in tissues in normal conditions is low. However, it rises on some developmental stages. For example, mouse and human CYP1A1 are highly expressed during early embryonic development. In the mouse embryos, CYP1A1 is expressed in the ectoderm at E7 gestational day and also during organogenesis in the heart at E8, hindbrain at E9, kidney at E12 and liver at E12.5 gestational day (Campbell et al., 2005; Ronis and, Cunny, 2008). Later, it returns to a barely detectable level later. This fact implies the existence of molecular mechanisms repressing expression of *CYP1A1* gene. It is known that the amount of AhR protein might influence transcription of *CYP1A1.* In addition, CYP1A1 expression may be downregulated by other transcription factors independently from AhR. Known molecular mechanisms responsible for the negative regulation of AhR and AhR-dependent genes are described below.

AhR expression depends on many factors of exogenous and endogenous origin. They are: AhR ligands and other xenobiotics, hormones, growth factors, cytokines, tumor growth, cell differentiation, age and others (Harper et al., 2006). AhR ligands decrease AhR protein levels by the negative feedback principle via proteasome degradation (Pollenz and Buggy, 2006). It is shown that TCDD shortens the half-life ($t_{1/2}$) and reduces the amount of AhR protein. Unliganded, cytoplasmic AhR is a stable protein with $t_{1/2}$ equal to 28 h. TCDD activation shortens the half-life period of AhR to to 3 h (Ma and Baldwin, 2000). The 26S proteasome inhibitors block this effect. Thus, the treatment with AhR ligands causes the acceleration of AhR protein degradation by proteasomes resulting in the negative regulation of AhR-dependent signal transduction pathway. The fact that a similar effect was not shown for Arnt, suggests that AhR, but not Arnt, interacts with the components of the ubiquitin-proteasome pathway. It has been shown that xenobiotic-activated AhR is degraded in the cytoplasm after being exported from the nucleus (Santiago-Josefat, 2001). Translocation from the cytosol is sufficient to trigger AhR degradation (Davarinos and Pollenz, 1999; Santiago-Josefat, 2001). The proteasomal degradation of AhR involves ubiquitination of AhR. It was demonstrated that TCDD induces ubiquitination of the AhR protein. Degradation through the ubiquitin-proteasome pathway requires the presence of a specific structural element called degron which is recognized by the ubiquitin-conjugating enzyme. It was shown that the C-terminal part of AhR which contains transactivation domains is important for the degradation of TCDD-activated AhR. It suggests that the transactivation domains function as a degron (Ma and Baldwin, 2000).

Negative regulation of the AhR-dependent signaling might also be mediated by AhR repressor (AhRR). This protein competes with AhR for binding to Arnt and forms heterodimers that are capable to bind to XRE, but do not stimulate the transcription of correspondent genes. Activation of AhRR expression occurs through the AhR-dependent signal transduction pathway. AhRR and AhR constitute a regulatory loop: the heterodimer AhR/Arnt activates AhRR expression. Expressed AhRR inhibits the function of AhR (Karchner et al, 2002; Zudaire et al, 2008).

Other proteins involved in the repression and termination of AhR signaling are AINT and ADPF. AINT (Arnt interacting protein), binds to Arnt and changes its cellular localization. According to Harper (Harper et al., 2006), in normal conditions, Arnt has nuclear localization, however, overexpression of AINT is accompanied by the decrease of nuclear levels of Arnt and the appearance of the proportional amount of Arnt in cytosol. ADPF (AhR degradation promoting factor) is the protein with an unknown function which is involved in the ubiquitin-dependent proteasomal degradation of AhR (Harper et al., 2006).

The function of AhR might be modulated (activated or inhibited) by a number of co-activators/co-repressors involved in the regulation of the AhR-dependent signal transduction pathway. AhR interacts with other transcription factors and multiple signaling molecules, such as NF-1 (nuclear factor 1), ERα (estrogen receptor-α), NF-κB (nuclear factor-kB), Mybbp1a (Myb-binding protein 1a), Nedd8 (neurally expressed developmentally down-regulated protein 8), Rb (retinoblastoma protein), Sp1 transcription factor, kinases, histone acetylating proteins and others (Harper et al., 2006).

Regulation of AhR and Arnt activities by protein kinases was described in detail in the chapter above called "AhR structure, function and signaling. Mechanism of CYP1A induction".

AhR regulation might be mediated via other signaling cascades. It was shown that components of the endocrine system influence the levels of AhR protein and mRNA. For example, in the liver of hypophysis-ectomized rats, the level of AhR protein was significantly decreased. This resulted in reduced binding of radioactively-labeled ligand to the cytosolic proteins. In this experiment, the changes in AHR protein level were not accompanied by the decrease of AhR and Arnt mRNAs and CYP1A1 activity. This indicates that the pituitary factor(s) regulates hepatic AHR expression on the protein level (Timsit et al., 2002).

The cross-talk between AhR and glucocorticoid receptor was demonstrated. In particular, synthetic glucocorticoid dexamethasone suppressed the expression of AhR and its target genes including CYP1A1 in cell culture. AhR acts synergistically with an activated glucocorticoid receptor (GR). AhR functionally interacts with GR and this leads to the further promotion of transactivation activity of the GR and an inhibition of transactivation activity of AhR (Sterling and Bresnick, 1996).

The inflammation factors also suppress AhR function. The potential molecular mechanism of this phenomenon might be related to the activation of a NF-κB-dependent signal transduction pathway since it was shown that NF-κB is able to bind to AhR. This results in the formation of an inactive complex and leads to mutual repression of both signaling cascades. Also, AhR and NF-κB are competitors for their common co-activators SRC1 and p300/CBP co-integrator proteins (Tian et al., 1999). NF-κB/AhR interaction converges at the level of transcription: NF-κB activation suppresses CYP1A1 expression by inhibiting histone H4 acetylation at CYP1A1 promoter (Ke et al., 2001). Many physiological functions such as immune system activation, skin differentiation, cell proliferation that are adversely affected by TCDD are regulated by NF-κB. It was demonstrated that TCDD activates NF-κB by AhR-independent mechanisms. Recently, evidences demonstrating that AhR and NF-κB interact and transcriptionally modulate each other were published (Tian et al., 2002).

Inhibition of CYP1A1 expression might also occur on the level of *CYP1A1* gene independently from AhR. A negative regulatory element (NRE) was found in the 5' region of CYP1A1. In mouse and human hepatoma cells transiently transfected with the construct, containing reporter gene under the control of different variants of CYP1A1 promoter, the removal of NRE from the 5'-region resulted in significantly increased activity of the reporter gene (Sterling et al., 1993). NRE contains binding sites at -808 to -788 bp position for at least three different proteins. One of the proteins binding to this regulatory region was identified as Oct-1. It was shown that Oct-1 binds to the 5′-upstream region of the *CYP1A1* and negatively regulates the expression of the correspondent gene. In addition, hyperexpression of Oct-1 causes a decrease of CYP1A1 expression (Sterling et al., 1993; Bhat et al., 1996; Sterling and Bresnick. 1996) as was shown using reporter-gene-based system. At the same time, the presence of high levels of Oct-1 did not influence the expression of the reporter gene under the control of promoter with mutant NRE region.

The protein C/EBPβ, a member of C/EBPs transcription factor's family (CCAA/enhancer binding proteins) was described as a factor that is involved in the negative regulation of CYP1A1 expression (Dale and Eltom, 2006). See the following chapter for details.

THE INHIBITION OF PAH-INDUCED CYP1A1 ACTIVATION

The number of studies devoted to the reduction of AhR and AhR targets hyperactivation has significantly risen during the last few years. Molecular mechanisms underlying the inhibition of PAH effects by other chemicals are described below. A separate sub-chapter is devoted to the antagonism of classic and weak CYP1A1 activators.

Negative Regulation of PAH-Induced CYP1A1 by Oxidative Processes

Oxidative processes might also affect activity of CYP1A1. It might occur on transcriptional, translational and post-translational levels. In mouse hepatoma Hepa-1c1c7 cells 1-nitropyrene, the member of nitro-PAHs, in combination with BP, decreased the level of BP-DNA adducts in a dose-dependent manner and enhanced CYP1A1 protein degradation (Cherng et al., 2006). Since these processes were accompanied by a higher production of reactive oxigene species (ROS) observed in binary mixture of BP and 1-nitropyrene in comparison with BP alone, authors suggested that the decrease of CYP1A1 protein levels in this case was attributed to the oxidative damage of protein by free radicals (Cherng et al., 2006).

It is shown that heavy metals modulate TCDD-induced CYP1A1 activity in human hepatoma HepG2 cells: arsenite (III) down-regulates TCDD-induced CYP1A1 activity, *CYP1A1* mRNA and protein level at the transcriptional and post-translational levels. Authors suggested that down-regulation of CYP1A1 by arsenite (III) was mediated by heme oxygenase-1 (HO-1) via an unidentified mechanism. Their conclusions were based on the following facts: (i) arsenite (III) increased HO-1 expression and this coincided with the decrease of CYP1A1 activity; (ii) competitive inhibitor of HO-1, tin mesoporphyrin, caused a partial restoration of the inhibition of TCDD-mediated induction of CYP1A1 by arsenite (III) (Anwar-Mohamed and El-Kadi, 2010). Exposure to mercury (Hg2+) or lead (Pb2+) also significantly decreased the activity of TCDD-induced CYP1A1, however, the protein and mRNA levels of the correspondent gene remained unchanged. It was postulated that the ability of both Hg2+ and Pb2+ to induce the expression of HO-1, a rate-limiting enzyme of heme degradation, could lead to the decrease of CYP1A1 activity levels (Korashy and El-Kadi, 2008).

Vanadium (5+) down-regulates TCDD-induced CYP1A1 activity, *CYP1A1* mRNA and protein levels in Hepa 1c1c7 cells through a transcriptional mechanism and in the human hepatoma HepG2 cells via transcriptional, post-transcriptional and post-translational mechanisms. Treatment of the cells with Va^{5+} did not ater the HO-1 expression. Instead, V5+ was found to induce the expression of Hif1α. Authors suggest that since Hif1α and AhR share the same dimerization partner Arnt, hypoxia might inhibit TCDD-mediated induction of CYP1A1 expression because of the competition between Hif1α and the AhR for Arnt (Abdelhamid et al., 2010).

The Inhibition of PAH-Induced CYP1A1 by Weak AhR Ligands / CYP1A Inducers

Competition for the Active Center of AhR

Some naturally-occurring polyphenols are able to down-regulate the effects of "classic" AhR ligands. It was shown that polyphenols directly inhibit CYP1A1 activity (Wen et al., 2010) and at least some of them demonstrated a competitive type of inhibition of CYP1A1 transcription (Kang et al., 1999; Wen et al., 2010). The extracts from black tea containing theaflavins also inhibited the binding of AhR to TCDD and AhR/Arnt complex to DNA (Fukuda et al., 2005). 6,2',4'-Trimethoxyflavone was able to displace PAHs fron AhR and thus, repress AhR-mediated gene induction (Murray et al., 2010). Curcumin was demonstrated to inhibit TCDD-induced CYP1A1 activity. It is known that this molecule is able to compete with TCDD for the active center of AhR, however, the proposed mechanism of CYP1A1 inhibition in this case is different and is associated with the phosphorylation of AhR. Details are described below.

Inhibition of the AhR and/or Arnt Phosphorylation

TCDD-induced DNA-binding activity of the AhR/Arnt heterodimer might be inhibited via the suppression of AhR and/or Arnt phosphorylation. This mechanism was described for curcumin which binds to a ligand-binding domain of the AhR. In untreated cells, curcumin stimulates AhR translocation to the nuclei and promotes its heterodimerization with Arnt, however, resulting heterodimers have significantly reduced ability to bind to XRE and stimulate CYP1A1 expression in comparison with the ones formed in the response to PAHs. In the case of co-treatment, curcumin promoted TCDD-activated AhR translocation to the nuclei but suppressed the formation of AhR/Arnt heterodimers, their binding to DNA and CYP1A1 expression induced by TCDD. Authors suggested that these effects of curcumin were attributed to the inhibition of AhR and Arnt phosphorylation. Proposed kinase involved in the process was PKC, because (i) curcumin dose-dependently inhibited its activity (ii) inhibitor of PKC also interfered with TCDD-stimulated formation of active DNA-binding heterodimers. It was reported that XRE-binding would require the phosphorylation of both AhR and Arnt, while for the formation of a heterodimer of these proteins, Arnt phosphorylation is sufficient. The main hypothesis is that the AhR translocated into the nucleus by curcumin promotes the formation of heterodimers lacking XRE-binding activity (Nishiumi et al., 2007).

According to the data of Mukai and co-authors (Mukai et al., 2010), flavones and flavonols suppress TCDD-induced dissociation of AhR and its partners (the structure of AhR cytosolic complex is described in details in the chapter "CYP1A induction mechanism. AhR structure, function and signaling"), reduce AhR nuclear translocation, the level of AhR and Arnt phosphorylation and AhR/Arnt complex formation in mouse hepatoma Hepa-1c1c7 cells.

Activation of the Transcription Factors Uppressing CYP1A1 Expression

Overexpression of the transcription factor C/EBPβ completely blocks the induction of CYP1A1 by 3-MC. Putative C/EBP binding site was identified in the CYP1A1 promoter region. This mechanism might be utilized by oltipraz, a cancer chemopreventive agent and anti-parasytic drug capable to inhibit the induction of CYP1A1 by 3-MC. It was demonstrated that this drug was also able to activate C/EBPβ (Cho and Kim, 2003). In addition, capsaicin, a component of chili peppers, inhibited CYP1A1 expression through C/EBPβ-mediated mechanism (Han et al., 2011).

Naturally-Occurring Compounds Down-regulating PAH-Induced CYP1A1 Induction by Unknown Mechanisms

Retinoids are thought to exert their effects on CYP1A1 through the cross-talk between AhR-dependent signal transduction pathway and retinoic acid-signaling pathway. The ability of retinoids to inhibit PAH-induced CYP1A1 induction and enzymatic activity was shown *in vivo* and *in vitro*.

In vitro, inhibitory ability of the following retinoids: all-trans-retinol, all-transretinal, all-trans-retinoic acid, and retinol-palmitate on CYP1A1 activity induced by PAHs was demonstrated in 1999 by Huang and co-authors and Inouye and co-authors (Inouye et al., 1999; Huang et al., 1999). They demonstrated that these compounds competitively inhibit CYP1A1 activity in the reconstituted system containing the microsomal fraction prepared from the recombinant Saccharomyces cerevisiae cells producing rat P4501A1 and yeast NADPH-P450 reductase (Inouye et al., 1999).

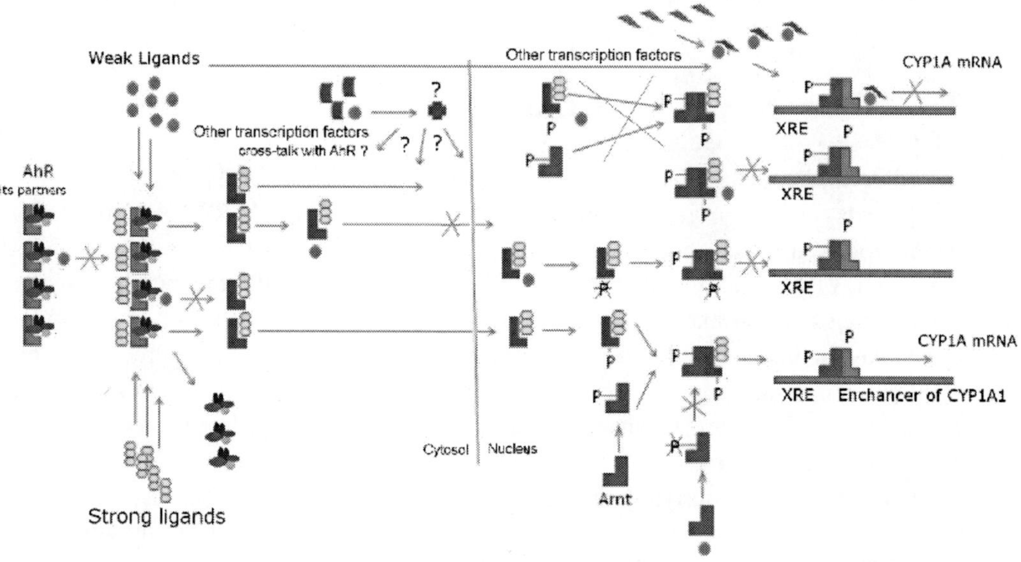

Figure 5. Possible mechanisms of inhibition of the AhR-dependent signal transduction pathway by weak AhR ligands. - Strong ligand; - Weak ligand; - Unactive AhR in complex with its protein partners; - Activated AhR; - Arnt; P - phosphorylated protein; → active process; - process is blocked; XRE – xenobiotic responsive element, AhR- aryl hydrocarbon receptor; Arnt - Ah receptor nuclear translocator.

In vivo, effects of vitamin A on CYP1A1 activity, *CYP1A1* mRNA levels and protein levels in the TCDD-treated mice's liver was shown by Yang and co-authors in 2005 (Yang et al., 2005). In the last work, the reduction of the liver damage, CYP1A1 activity, *CYP1A1* and *AhR* expression levels was observed in the liver of the rat receiving the combination of TCDD and vitamin A in comparison with animals treated with TCDD alone. Also, retinal and retinol competitively inhibited BP metabolism in 3-MC-treated rats (Huang et al., 1999). It is unclear, if vitamin A effects on CYP1A1 are attributed to the cross-talk between AhR-dependent signal transduction pathway and retinoic acid-signaling pathway or by other mechanisms.

5,7-Dimethoxyflavone, downregulates BP-induced CYP1A1 activity, *CYP1A1* mRNA levels, protein expression and DNA binding in Hep G2 cells; mechanism of this effect is not known (Wen et al., 2005).

Our previous data (Sidorova and Grishanova, 2005) shows that rats treated with both BP (BP) and alpha-tocopherol had significantly lower CYP1A1 activity in the liver in comparison with animals treated with BP alone. In addition, alpha-tocopherol inhibits

CYP1A1 activity *in vitro* in the microsomes isolated from the liver of BP-treated animals. We assume, that the inhibition of BP-induced CYP1A1 activity by alpha-tocopherol is mediated at the post-translational level because the level of CYP1A1 protein in the liver is the same in both treatment groups: receiving BP and alpha-tocopherol together and BP alone. This inhibitiory effect of alpha-tocopheral was not attributed to ROS production, since oxidative stress markers were significantly reduced in the liver of animals treated with vitamin E. We think that alpha-tocopherol might directly inhibit CYP1A1 activity *in vivo* in rat liver, as it was shown on rat hepatic microsomes *in vitro*.

CONCLUSION

According to the general belief, most if not all adverse effects of TCDD-like and PAH-like compounds on the organism are mediated by AhR and AhR-dependent proteins (Birnbaum, 2004). It occurs on two levels: via the formation of highly reactive metabolites produced by CYP1A and via interference of activated AhR with the number of other regulatory proteins which may cause various disorders. Scientists and health care providers started to make attempts to neutralize toxic effects of dioxins some time ago. Previously, most of the actions aimed at symptomatic treatment of chloracne, the main syndrome of acute poisoning with dioxins were taken. To reduce intoxication, anti-inflammatory agents and sorbents promoting the removal of dioxin from the body were used. After elucidation of molecular mechanism underlying the effects of dioxin on the organism, including participation of AhR and the induction of CYP1A, scientists began to try to influence these disorders at the molecular level. Firstly, the efforts were concentrated on the reduction of oxidative stress, which appeared as a result of the ROS generation by activated CYP1A (Alsharif and Hassoun, 2004; Hassoun et al., 2004). Now, the knowledge about molecular mechanisms of AhR normal function and consequences of AhR activation continues to expand rapidly. These data allow searching for novel, more effective ways to prevent dioxin-caused disorders.

PAHs are presented in emissions from thermal power generation, in tobacco smoke and in car exhaust. The air pollution with dangerous compounds including PAH in big sites is getting higher every year. Thus, the risk of exposure to these chemicals is also increasing. Contact with low doses of PAHs does not lead to acute poisoning and that is why it is asymptomatic, however, most likely it is not harmless. This is supported by epidemiological data demonstrating an association between the risk of developing cancer and exposure to PAHs. Thus, identification and characterization of novel molecules preventing and reducing PAH-induced effects is very important.

It is clear that the reduction of BP-DNA adducts level and CYP1A expression caused by the combination of different "strong" and dangerous AhR activators and heavy metals is an interesting fact, but it is unlikely that these data can be used to develop treatments and / or prevention of dioxin-related disorders in humans. From a therapeutic point of view, the more interesting substances interfering with PAH effects and inhibiting AhR-dependent signal transduction pathways are physiological compounds such as vitamins and food components. These molecules are proven to be non-toxic for mammals by many years of use and can represent a novel approach to combat dioxin toxicity on molecular level. It is worthy to note, that some of these molecules were shown to prevent PAH-induced carcinogenesis, however, the basis for such effect had not been known [74, 28]. Recent studies reviewed in this paper shed light on potential molecular mechanisms underlying this phenomenon. However, in spite of multiple efforts, in many cases, the mode of action of these compounds in context of their antagonism with PAH remains unknown or not fully understood and thus needs to be investigated further.

REFERENCES

Abdelhamid, G; Anwar-Mohamed, A; Badary, OA; Moustafa, AA; El-Kadi, AO. Transcriptional and post-transcriptional regulation of CYP1A1 by vanadium in human hepatoma HepG2 cells. Cell Biol Toxicol, 2010, 26, 421-34.

Adachi, J; Mori, Y; Matsui, S; Takigami, H; Fujino, J; Kitagawa, H; Miller, CA 3rd; Kato, T; Saeki, K; Matsuda, T. Indirubin and indigo are potent aryl hydrocarbon receptor ligands present in human urine. J Biol Chem, 2001, 276, 31475-8.

Allen, SW; Mueller, L; Williams, SN; Quattrochi, LC; Raucy, J. The use of a high-volume screening procedure to assess the effects of dietary flavonoids on human cyp1a1 expression. Drug Metab Dispos, 2001, 29, 1074-9.

Alsharif, NZ; Hassoun, EA. Protective effects of vitamin A and vitamin E succinate against 2,3,7,8-tetrachlorodibenzo-p-dioxin (TCDD)-induced body wasting, hepatomegaly, thymic atrophy, production of reactive oxygen species and DNA damage in C57BL/6J mice. Basic Clin Pharmacol Toxicol., 2004, 95, 131-8.

Anwar-Mohamed, A; El-Kadi, AO. Arsenite down-regulates cytochrome P450 1A1 at the transcriptional and post-translational levels in human HepG2 cells. Free Radic Biol Med, 2010, 48, 1399-409.

Astorg, P; Gradelet, S; Leclerc, J; Siess, MH. Effects of provitamin A or non-provitamin A carotenoids on liver xenobiotic-metabolizing enzymes in mice. Nutr Cancer, 1997, 27, 245-9.

Backlund, M; Ingelman-Sundberg, M. Different structural requirements of the ligand binding domain of the aryl hydrocarbon receptor for high- and low-affinity ligand binding and receptor activation. Mol Pharmacol, 2004, 65, 416-25.

Beischlag, TV; Luis, Morales J; Hollingshead, BD; Perdew, GH. The aryl hydrocarbon receptor complex and the control of gene expression. Crit Rev Eukaryot Gene Expr, 2008, 18, 207-50.

Bhat, R; Weaver, JA; Sterling, KM; Bresnick, E. Nuclear transcription factor Oct-1 binds to the 5'-upstream region of CYP1A1 and negatively regulates its expression. Int J Biochem Cell Biol, 1996, 28, 217-27.

Birnbaum, LS. The mechanism of dioxin toxicity: relationship to risk assessment. Environ Health Perspect, 1994, 102, 157-67.

Bohonowych, JE; Denison, MS. Persistent binding of ligands to the aryl hydrocarbon receptor. Toxicol Sci, 2007, 98, 99-109.

Campbell, SJ; Henderson, CJ; Anthony, DC; Davidson, D; Clark, AJ; Wolf, CR. The murine Cyp1a1 gene is expressed in a restricted spatial and temporal pattern during embryonic development. J Biol Chem, 2005, 280, 5828-35.

Carver, LA; Jackiw, V; Bradfield, CA. The 90-kDa heat shock protein is essential for Ah receptor signaling in a yeast expression system. J Biol Chem, 1994, 269, 30109-12.

Céspedes, MA; Galindo, MI; Couso, JP. Dioxin toxicity in vivo results from an increase in the dioxin-independent transcriptional activity of the aryl hydrocarbon receptor. PLoS One, 2010, 5, e15382.

Cherng, SH; Hsu, SL; Yang, JL; Yu, CT; Lee, H. Suppressive effect of 1-nitropyrene on benzo[a]pyrene-induced CYP1A1 protein expression in HepG2 cells. Toxicol Lett, 2006, 161, 236-43.

Cho, IJ; Kim, SG. Oltipraz inhibits 3-methylcholanthrene induction of CYP1A1 by CCAAT/enhancer-binding protein activation. J Biol Chem, 2003, 278, 44103-12.

Ciolino, HP; Daschner, PJ; Wang, TT; Yeh, GC. Effect of curcumin on the aryl hydrocarbon receptor and cytochrome P450 1A1 in MCF-7 human breast carcinoma cells. Biochem Pharmacol, 1998, 56, 197-206.

Ciolino, HP; Daschner, PJ; Yeh, GC. Dietary flavonols quercetin and kaempferol are ligands of the aryl hydrocarbon receptor that affect CYP1A1 transcription differentially. Biochem J, 1999, 340, 715-22.

Dale, Y; Eltom, SE. The induction of CYP1A1 by oltipraz is mediated through calcium-dependent-calpain. Toxicol Lett. 2006,166, 150-9.

Davarinos, NA; Pollenz, RS. Aryl hydrocarbon receptor imported into the nucleus following ligand binding is rapidly degraded via the cytosplasmic proteasome following nuclear export. J Biol Chem, 1999, 274, 28708-15.

Delescluse, C; Lemaire, G; de Sousa, G; Rahmani, R. Is CYP1A1 induction always related to AHR signaling pathway? Toxicology, 2000, 153, 73-82.

Denison, MS; Nagy, SR. Activation of the aryl hydrocarbon receptor by structurally diverse exogenous and endogenous chemicals. Annu Rev Pharmacol Toxicol, 2003, 43, 309-34.

Enan, E; Matsumura, F. Identification of c-Src as the integral component of the cytosolic Ah receptor complex, transducing the signal of 2,3,7,8-tetrachlorodibenzo-p-dioxin (TCDD) through the protein phosphorylation pathway. Biochem Pharmacol, 1996, 52, 1599-1612.

Fujii-Kuriyama, Y; Kawajiri, K; Molecular mechanisms of the physiological functions of the aryl hydrocarbon (dioxin) receptor, a multi-functional regulator that senses and responds to environmental stimuli. Proc Jpn Acad Ser B Phys Biol Sci, 2010, 86, 40-53.

Fukuda, I; Sakane, I; Yabushita, Y; Sawamura, S; Kanazawa, K; Ashida, H. Black tea theaflavins suppress dioxin-induced transformation of the aryl hydrocarbon receptor. Biosci Biotechnol Biochem, 2005, 69, 883-90.

Gambone, CJ; Hutcheson, JM; Gabriel, JL; Beard, RL; Chandraratna, RA; Soprano, KJ; Soprano, DR. Unique property of some synthetic retinoids: activation of the aryl hydrocarbon receptor pathway. Mol Pharmacol, 2002, 61, 334-42.

Garg, R; Gupta, S; Maru, GB. Dietary curcumin modulates transcriptional regulators of phase I and phase II enzymes in benzo[a]pyrene-treated mice: mechanism of its anti-initiating action. Carcinogenesis, 2008, 29, 1022-32.

Grishanova, AIu; Zueva, TV. [Bilirubin as an endogenous intermediary in the activation of CYP1A1 expression upon exposure to ultrasound]. Vopr Med Khim, 2000, 46, 117-26.

Gunton, JE; Kulkarni, RN; Yim, S; Okada, T; Hawthorne, WJ; Tseng, YH; Roberson, RS; Ricordi, C; O'Connell, PJ; Gonzalez, FJ; Kahn, CR. Loss of ARNT/HIF1beta mediates altered gene expression and pancreatic-islet dysfunction in human type 2 diabetes. Cell, 2005, 122, 337-49.

Han, EH; Hwang, YP; Kim, HG; Choi, JH; Park, BH; Song, GY; Lee, GW; Jeong, TC; Jeong, HG CCAAT/enhancer-binding protein β activation by capsaicin contributes to the regulation of CYP1A1 expression, mediated by the aryl hydrocarbon receptor. Br J Pharmacol, 2011, Jan 21. doi: 10.1111/j.1476-5381.2011.01232.x. [Epub ahead of print]

Harper, PA; Riddick, DS; Okey, AB. Regulating the regulator: factors that control levels and activity of the aryl hydrocarbon receptor. Biochem Pharmacol, 2006, 72, 267-279.

Harstad, EB; Guite, CA; Thomae, TL; Bradfield, CA. Liver deformation in Ahr-null mice: evidence for aberrant hepatic perfusion in early development. Mol Pharmacol, 2006, 69, 1534-41.

Hassoun, EA; Vodhanel, J; Abushaban, A; The modulatory effects of ellagic acid and vitamin E succinate on TCDD-induced oxidative stress in different brain regions of rats after subchronic exposure. J Biochem Mol Toxicol, 2004, 18, 196-203.

Heath-Pagliuso, S; Rogers, WJ; Tullis, K; Seidel, SD; Cenijn, PH; Brouwer, A; Denison, MS. Activation of the Ah receptor by tryptophan and tryptophan metabolites. Biochemistry, 1998, 37, 11508-15.

Helferich, WG; Denison, MS. Ultraviolet photoproducts of tryptophan can act as dioxin agonists. Ultraviolet Mol Pharmacol, 1991, 40, 674-8.

Hernández-Ochoa, I; Karman, BN; Flaws, JA. The role of the aryl hydrocarbon receptor in the female reproductive system. Biochem Pharmacol, 2009, 77, 547-59.

Huang, DY; Ohnishi, T; Jiang, H; Furukawa, A; Ichikawa, Y. Inhibition by retinoids of benzo(A)pyrene metabolism catalyzed by 3- methylcholanthrene-induced rat cytochrome P-450 1A1. Metabolism, 1999, 48, 689–692.

Inouye, K; Mae, T; Kondo, S; Ohkawa, H. Inhibitory effects of vitamin A and vitamin K on rat cytochrome P4501A1-dependent monooxygenase activity. Biochem Biophys Res Commun, 1999, 262, 565–569.

Kang, ZC; Tsai, SJ; Lee, H. Quercetin inhibits benzo[a]pyrene-induced, D.N.A adducts in human Hep G2 cells by altering cytochome P-450 1A1 gene expression. Nutr Cancer, 1999, 35, 175-179.

Karchner, SI; Franks, DG; Powell, WH; Hahn, ME. Regulatory interactions among three members of the vertebrate aryl hydrocarbon receptor family: AHR repressor, AHR1, and AHR2. Biol Chem, 2002, 277, 6949-59.

Kazlauskas, A; Poellinger, L; Pongratz, I. The immunophilin-like protein XAP2 regulates ubiquitination and subcellular localization of the dioxin receptor. J Biol Chem, 2000, 275, 41317-24.

Ke, S; Rabson, AB; Germino, JF; Gallo, MA; Tian, Y. Mechanism of suppression of cytochrome P-450 1A1 expression by tumor necrosis factor-alpha and lipopolysaccharide. J Biol Chem, 2001, 26, 39638-44

Korashy, HM; El-Kadi, AO. Modulation of TCDD-mediated induction of cytochrome P450 1A1 by mercury, lead, and copper in human HepG2 cell line. Toxicol In Vitro, 2008, 22, 154-8.

Lemaire, G; Delescluse, C; Pralavorio, M; Ledirac, N; Lesca, P; Rahmani, R. The role of protein tyrosine kinases in CYP1A1 induction by omeprazole and thiabendazole in rat hepatocytes. Life Sci. 2004, 74, 2265-78.

Levine, SL; Perdew, GH. Aryl hydrocarbon receptor (AhR)/AhR nuclear translocator (ARNT) activity is unaltered by phosphorylation of a periodicity/ARNT/single-minded (PAS)-region serine residue. Mol Pharmacol, 2001, 59, 557-566.

Long, WP; Chen, X; Perdew, GH. Protein kinase C modulates aryl hydrocarbon receptor nuclear translocator protein-mediated transactivation potential in a dimer context. J Biol Chem, 1999, 274, 12391-400.

Ma, C; Marlowe, JL; Puga, A. The aryl hydrocarbon receptor at the crossroads of multiple signaling pathways. EXS, 2009, 99, 231-257.

Ma, Q. Induction of CYP1A1. The AhR/DRE paradigm: transcription, receptor regulation, and expanding biological roles. Curr Drug Metab, 2001, 2, 149-164.

Ma, Q; Baldwin, KT. 2,3,7,8-tetrachlorodibenzo-p-dioxin-induced degradation of aryl hydrocarbon receptor (AhR) by the ubiquitin-proteasome pathway. Role of the transcription activaton and DNA binding of AhR. J Biol Chem, 2000, 275, 8432-8.

Ma, Q; Dong, L; Whitlock, JP Jr. Transcriptional activation by the mouse Ah receptor. Interplay between multiple stimulatory and inhibitory functions. J Biol Chem, 1995, 270, 12697-703.

Machemer, DE; Tukey, RH. The role of protein kinase C in regulation of TCDD-mediated CYP1A1 gene expression. Toxicol Sci, 2005, 87, 27-37.

Marinković, N; Pašalić, D; Ferenčak, G; Gršković, B; Stavljenić Rukavina, A. Dioxins and human toxicity. Arh Hig Rada Toksikol, 2010, 61, 445-53.

Minsavage, GD; Park, SK; Gasiewicz, TA. The aryl hydrocarbon receptor (AhR) tyrosine 9, a residue that is essential for AhR DNA binding activity, is not a phosphoresidue but augments AhR phosphorylation. Biol Chem, 2004, 279, 20582-93.

Mukai, R; Shirai, Y; Saito, N; Fukuda, I; Nishiumi, S; Yoshida, K; Ashida, H. Suppression mechanisms of flavonoids on aryl hydrocarbon receptor-mediated signal transduction. Arch Biochem Biophys, 2010, 501, 134-41.

Murphy, KA; Quadro, L; White, LA. The intersection between the aryl hydrocarbon receptor (AhR)- and retinoic acid-signaling pathways. Vitam Horm, 2007, 75, 33-67.

Murray, IA; Flaveny, CA; DiNatale, BC; Chairo, CR; Schroeder, JC; Kusnadi, A; Perdew, GH. Antagonism of aryl hydrocarbon receptor signaling by 6,2',4'-trimethoxyflavone. Pharmacol Exp Ther, 2010, 332, 135-44.

Nguyen, LP; Bradfield, CA. The search for endogenous activators of the aryl hydrocarbon receptor. Chem Res Toxicol, 2008, 21, 102-16..

Nishiumi, S; Yoshida, K; Ashida, H. Curcumin suppresses the transformation of an aryl hydrocarbon receptor through its phosphorylation. Arch Biochem Biophys, 2007, 466, 267-73.

Pelclová, D; Urban, P; Preiss, J; Lukás, E; Fenclová, Z; Navrátil, T; Dubská, Z; Senholdová, Z. Adverse health effects in humans exposed to 2,3,7,8-tetrachlorodibenzo-p-dioxin (TCDD). Rev Environ Health, 2006, 21, 119-38.

Petrulis, JR; Perdew, GH. The role of chaperone proteins in the aryl hydrocarbon receptor core complex. Chem Biol Interact, 2002, 141, 25-40.

Phelan, D; Winter, GM; Rogers, WJ; Lam, JC; Denison, MS. Activation of the Ah receptor signal transduction pathway by bilirubin and biliverdin. Arch Biochem Biophys. 1998, 357, 155-63.

Pollenz, RS; Buggy, C. Ligand-dependent and -independent degradation of the human aryl hydrocarbon receptor (hAHR) in cell culture models. Chem Biol Interact, 2006, 164, 49-59.

Quattrochi, LC; Vu, T; Tukey, RH. The human CYP1A2 gene and induction by 3-methylcholanthrene. A region of DNA that supports AH-receptor binding and promoter-specific induction. J Biol Chem, 1994, 269, 6949-54.

Raffalli-Mathieu, F; Geneste, O; Lang, MA. Characterization of two nuclear proteins that interact with cytochrome P-450 1A2 mRNA. Regulation of RNA binding and possible role in the expression of the Cyp1a2 gene. Eur J Biochem, 1997, 245, 17-24.

Ramadoss, P; Perdew, GH. The transactivation domain of the Ah receptor is a key determinant of cellular localization and ligand-independent nucleocytoplasmic shuttling properties. Biochemistry, 2005, 44, 11148-59.

Ronis, MJJ; Cunny, HC. Developmental effects on xenobiotics metabolism. In: Smart RS, Hodgson E. editors. Molecular and Biochemical Toxicology, 4th Edition. New Jersey: John Wiley & Sons, Inc; 2008; 257-272.

Rüegg, J; Swedenborg, E; Wahlström, D; Escande, A; Balaguer, P; Pettersson, K; Pongratz, I. The transcription factor aryl hydrocarbon receptor nuclear translocator functions as an estrogen receptor beta-selective co-activator, and its recruitment to alternative pathways mediates anti-estrogenic effects of dioxin. Mol Endocrinol, 2008, 22, 304-16.

Santiago-Josefat, B; Pozo-Guisado, E; Mulero-Navarro, S; Fernandez-Salguero, PM. Proteasome inhibition induces nuclear translocation and transcriptional activation of the dioxin receptor in mouse embryo primary fibroblasts in the absence of xenobiotics. Mol Cell Biol, 2001, 21, 1700-9.

Santiago-Josefat, BE; Pozo-Guisado, E; Mulero-Navarro, S; Fernandez-Salguero, PM. Proteasome inhibition induces nuclear translocation and transcriptional activation of the dioxin receptor in mouse embryo primary fibroblasts in the absence of xenobiotics. J Mol Cell Biol. 2001, 21, 1700–1709.

Savouret, JF; Antenos, M; Quesne, M; Xu, J; Milgrom, E; Casper, RF. 7-ketocholesterol is an endogenous modulator for the arylhydrocarbon receptor. J Biol Chem, 2001, 276, 3054-9.

Schrenk, D; Riebniger, D; Till, M; Vetter, S; Fiedler, HP. Tryptanthrins and other tryptophan-derived agonists of the dioxin receptor. Adv Exp Med Biol, 1999, 467, 403-8.

Seidel, SD; Winters, GM; Rogers, WJ; Ziccardi, MH; Li, V; Keser, B; Denison, MS. Activation of the Ah receptor signaling pathway by prostaglandins. J Biochem Mol Toxicol, 2001, 15, 187-96.

Sidorova, YA; Grishanova, AY. Inhibitory effect of alpha-tocopherol on benzo(a)pyrene-induced CYPA1 activity in rat liver. Bull Exp Biol Med, 2005, 140, 517-20.

Sidorova, YA; Grishanova, AY; Lyakhovich, VV. Rat hepatic CYP1A1 and CYP1A2 induction by menadione. Toxicol Lett, 2005, 155, 253-8.

Sidorova, YA; Grishanova, AY; Lyakhovich, VV. Transcriptional activation of cytochrome P450 1A1 with alpha-tocopherol. Bull Exp Biol Med, 2004, 138, 233-6.

Smith, GB; Harper, PA; Wong, JM; Lam, MS; Reid, KR; Petsikas, D; Massey, TE. Human lung microsomal cytochrome P4501A1 (CYP1A1) activities: impact of smoking status and CYP1A1, aryl hydrocarbon receptor, and glutathione S-transferase M1 genetic polymorphisms. Cancer Epidemiol Biomarkers Prev, 2001, 10, 839-53.

Soshilov, A; Denison, MS. Role of the Per/Arnt/Sim domains in ligand-dependent transformation of the aryl hydrocarbon receptor. J Biol Chem, 2008, 283, 32995-3005.

Sterling, K; Bresnick, E. Oct-1 transcription factor is a negative regulator of rat CYP1A1 expression via an octamer sequence in its negative regulatory element. Mol Pharmacol. 1996, 49, 329-37.

Sterling, K; Weaver, J; Ho, KL; Xu, LC; Bresnick, E. Rat CYP1A1 negative regulatory element: biological activity and interaction with a protein from liver and hepatoma cells. Mol Pharmacol, 1993, 44, 560-8.

Tian, Y; Ke, S; Denison, MS; Rabson, AB; Gallo, MA. Ah receptor and NF-kappaB interactions, a potential mechanism for dioxin toxicity. J Biol Chem, 1999, 274, 510-5.

Tian, Y; Rabson, AB; Gallo, MA. Ah receptor and NF-kappaB interactions: mechanisms and physiological implications. Chem Biol Interact. 2002, 141, 97-115.

Timsit, YE; Chia, FS; Bhathena, A; Riddick, DS. Aromatic hydrocarbon receptor expression and function in liver of hypophysectomized male rats. Toxicol Appl Pharmacol, 2002, 185, 136-45.

Wen, X; Walle, UK; Walle, T. 5,7-Dimethoxyflavone downregulates CYP1A1 expression and benzo[a]pyrene-induced DNA binding in Hep G2 cells. Carcinogenesis, 2005, 26, 803-9.

Whitlock, JPJr. Induction of cytochrome P4501A1. Annu Rev Pharmacol Toxicol, 1999, 39, 103-125.

Yang, YM; Huang, DY; Liu, GF; Zhong, JC; Du, K; Li, YF; Song, XH. Inhibitory effects of vitamin A on TCDD-induced cytochrome P-450 1A1 enzyme activity and expression. Toxicol Sci, 2005, 85, 727-34.

Zudaire, E; Cuesta, N; Murty, V; Woodson, K; Adams, L; Gonzalez, N; Martínez, A; Narayan, G; Kirsch, I; Franklin, W; Hirsch, F; Birrer, M; Cuttitta, F. The aryl hydrocarbon receptor repressor is a putative tumor suppressor gene in multiple human cancers. J Clin Invest, 2008, 118, 640-50.

In: Xenobiotics: New Research
Editors: Saul F. Castaneda and Mauro L. Emerson
ISBN: 978-1-61942-616-0

Chapter 3

Esposition of Marine Copepods to Organophosphorus Xenobiotics: Application of Acetylcholinesterase Biomarkers in the Laboratory

C. Agrone, M. G. Aluigi, G. L. Mariottini, E. Giacco, A. Somà, C. Falugi, and L. Pane
Dipteris University of Genova, Viale Benedetto XV 5, Genova, Italy

Abstract

Organophosphorus pesticides (OP) are dangerous xenobiotics for aquatic environments mainly because they can interact with all links of the food web inducing bioaccumulation and bioconcentration in organisms. In addition, they have an influence on the enzymes of the cholinergic system (acetylcholinesterase and pseudocholinesterase) of the organisms blocking their catalytic site and causing an excess of excitation of receptors for acetylcholine accumulation. The biomarkers, such as the evaluation of acetylcholinesterase (AChE) inhibition, provide an indication of the pollution level of the environment and are indicators of the ecotoxicological risk for exposed organisms. As small invertebrates are a fundamental link in the food web, the ecotoxicological risk evaluated on these organisms with the biomarker approach can be used as an early evidence of ecosystem damage. In this research copepods collected in the splashpools of the eastern coast of the Ligurian Sea and maintained in the laboratory were utilized as test-organisms. Aim of this work was to evaluate in copepods *Tigriopus fulvus* the effect of the exposition to the organophosphorus pesticide Malathion (Pestanal®) on the activity of AChE.

Introduction

In the last decades Ecotoxicology has assumed a remarkable importance in the scientific overview as a consequence of pollution problems caused mainly by the industrial development and by several human activities. As a matter of fact Ecotoxicology, studying the transformations of pollutants within the organisms and the transformed features of such substances after the release into the environment subsequent to excretion or to organism death, as well as the final fate in the environment and the final features of re-introduced compounds, makes up a new integrated applicative approach to Biology and to environmental Chemistry aimed to work out precautionary measures useful to counter the emergence of harmful effects (Vighi, 1989; Vismara, 1992; Carli *et al.*, 1998).

A lot of research have emphasized that chemical monitoring of environmental pollution is not sufficient to determine the environmental risk of pollutant mixtures; as a matter of fact, it takes the immediate occurrence of pollutants, but it is not able to assess their effects on organisms, being unaware of the synergies between the environmental compartments (Vighi, 1989; Vismara, 1992; Marchetti, 1993; ARPAL, 2004).

In the last years ecotoxicological tests, both in field and in the laboratory, have been increasingly employed as a method to flank the chemical assessment in the evaluation of environmental pollution, because they allow to quantify the potential environmental risk of chemicals, being also essential in the procedures to evaluate the risk for humans and for the environment (Oddo, 2001).

The test pertinent to the aquatic environments are carried out using organisms belonging to different trophic levels (primary producers, primary consumers, secondary consumers, decomposers). The choice of the test-species should be made considering different aspects of which the most important are: availability, easy breeding, sensitivity to toxicants and standardization of methods; in addition, a good knowledge of life cycle is essential (Vighi, 1989; Widdows, 1994; Carli *et al.*, 1998; Pane *et al.*, 2007).

Another supplementary approach used for the evaluation of toxic effects at different organization levels and in the environmental monitoring, concerns the evaluation of biological indicators of exposition, namely the biomarkers. These indicators have been evaluated in different organisms in relation to the exposition to different xenobiotics such as some non-essential heavy metals and diverse persistent organic compounds such as pesticides (NRC, 1989; Fossi, 1991; Bacci, 1994; Depledge, 1994; Dagnino *et al.*, 2007; Aluigi *et al.*, 2008).

The pesticides are harmful for the marine environment because they have an action on all levels of the trophic chain (Duursma & Marchand, 1974). Even though the spreading of pesticides in seawaters has been recently reduced (Powe *et al.*, 1999), owing to their persistence, and particularly to that of compounds used in the past, the problems linked to their occurrence have not been quite solved (Dahr *et al.*, 2004; Thiere & Schulz, 2004).

The studies concerning the toxicity of these substances on aquatic organisms (such as echinoderms and molluscs) are exhaustive, while those pertinent to other taxa are limited. Among freshwater species cladocerans *Daphnia magna* and *Ceriodaphnia dubia* and among marine crustaceans the brine shrimp *Artemia salina*, the mysid *Misidyopsis bahia* and the copepod *Acartia tonsa* are currently employed. Nevertheless, the utilization of such organisms suffers some problems mainly due to the low sensitivity of *A. salina* to xenobiotics and to the strong limitations to dispose *A. tonsa* e *M. bahia* in some zones such as in the Mediterranean region, where *Acartia tonsa* is not endemic, in fact it was known to occur only recently, and *Mysidopsis bahia* (also named *Americamysis bahia*) does not occur at all being typical of Atlantic American coasts and of the Gulf of Mexico (EPA, 2002). Furthermore, to date the studies of the effects on these crustaceans of organophosphorus pesticides, in terms of biomarkers, are quite occasional.

On this basis, aim of this work was to evaluate the effect of the exposition to the organophosphorus pesticide Malathion, Pestanal® on the activity of AChE of an emergent species eligible to play the role of test-species in ecotoxicology, namely the copepods *Tigriopus fulvus*, reared in laboratory conditions.

THE PESTICIDES AND THEIR EFFECTS

The knowledge of pollution sources and of their impact on the ecosystems is a subject of concern to achieve a better knowledge of the environmental responses to pollutants and to work out suitable prevention standards. The impact of these pollution sources on marine and freshwaters, such as the effects on water chemical composition (James *et al.*, 2005; Olson *et al.*, 2005) with consequent eutrophication and alterations of the food-web (Pretty *et al.*, 2003; Moss, 2004), biocide wash-out (Traas *et al.*, 2004; Christensen *et al.*, 2005), material suspension after soil erosion (Brodie & Mitchell, 2005), alteration of hydrological cycles (Williams & Aladin, 1991) and environmental physical changes (Raven *et al.*, 1998) is mainly due to anthropogenic causes.

Pesticides, being lipophilic and able to release residues, were shown to be among the most dangerous toxicants for aquatic ecosystems because they interfere with all links of the food-web (Duursma & Marchand, 1974) through two important mechanisms: bioconcentration (direct accumulation of chemicals from the environment) and biomagnification (increasing of the concentration of chemicals passing from a trophic level to the subsequent, due to the accumulation through the food-web); for this reason high concentrations of pollutants can be recorded in the top predators and also in humans (Fleeger *et al.*, 2003; Islam & Tanaka, 2004).

Pesticide dispersal in waters showed a remarkable decrease in the last years (Powe *et al.*, 1999); nevertheless, from published data it can be inferred that to date a lot of problems still subsist (Dahr *et al.*, 2004; Thiere & Schulz, 2004) because consistent remnants of biocides and pesticides released some decades ago still persist in waters, and are to date findable, for example, in Antarctica and presumptively can occur everywhere (Moss, 2008).

Pesticides are natural or synthetic compounds used to fight vegetal or animal pests able to damage crops (Carli *et al.*, 1998). According to the chemical structure pesticides are subdivided into categories; the action mechanism and the selectivity of the compound against the physiology of the target-organism are also due to the chemical structure. The persistence of pesticides in the environment differs according to their chemical characteristics and the degradation can be carried out by specific micro-organisms and also through the action of temperature or other physical agents.

In the past several pesticides were characterized by high environmental persistence, so that they were named "Persistent Organic Pollutants (POPs)". The POPs are chemicals determining remarkable risks for humans and for the environment because they persist into the environment, bioaccumulate into high lipid content tissues, pass from the mother to the foetus, are toxic and harmful both for the environment and humans, move with the wind, surface waters and marine currents covering huge distances.

Neurotoxic pesticides, and mainly organophosphates, are used worldwide to fight the diseases given by insects and small invertebrates. To date the modern insecticides are less persistent than those formerly used, but in order to do their function as soon as possible, they are provided with higher toxic features. From the literature organophosphates are known to produce disorders of the Central Nervous System, psychometric changes, disturbances of memory, anxiety and depression (Jamal *et al.*, 2002). In addition, organophosphates are lipophilic and are able to stay behind body fats exerting a chronic action. Neurotoxic pesticides have the cholinergic system and the neuromuscular system as a target; in particular, the toxic effects of these compounds are due to their capability to inhibit lytic enzymes of the cholinergic system, the acetylcholinesterase (AChE) and the pseudo-cholinesterase (pseudo-ChE).

The organophosphates bind to the AChE causing its irreversible inhibition (Sultatos, 1994) and an excess of excitation of the receptors for the acetylcholine (ACh) accumulation in the receptors themselves (Karczmar *et al.*, 1970). The accumulation of ACh in the receptors can cause both receptor desensitization (paradoxical effect) and increase of signal transmission.

In this research the ecotoxicity of the pesticide Malathion Pestanal®, still used with some restrictions, was evaluated. This compound was chosen because it is considered scarcely persistent (Kow=562, BCF=103), but highly effective on target organisms and consequently potentially harmful for the environment.

Malathion is a wide-spectrum insecticide and was among the first used organophosphates (from 1950) to control insects and fruit and vegetables pests (USEPA, 1988). It is a yellowish-transparent fluid poorly water-soluble (145 mg/l at 20 °C) and is miscible in several organic solvents (Hazardous Substances Data Bank, 2000). It is relatively resistant to the photolysis but it is hydrolized in alcaline conditions (USEPA, 2000a); the microbial metabolism is its main way of degradation in soils where the half-life time varies between 1 and 25 days (Hornsby *et al.*, 1999). Malathion is greatly movable and its short staying into the soil reduces the pollution of aquifers. The biodegradation and the pH affect greatly its persistence in surface waters: as a matter of fact, its degradation can amount to 75% after a week and 90% after two weeks in freshwaters (USEPA, 2000a); the vaporization is not significant (Howard, 1991).

Malathion is considered to be harmful (Xn), dangerous for the environment (N), harmful by ingestion (R22), highly toxic to aquatic organisms (R50/53). Studies considering the reproduction of mice along two generations did not show effects on fertility, but only weight decrease of adults (USEPA, 2000b); similar results were obtained as concerns the teratogenicity (Marrs, 1997; USEPA, 2000b).

On the contrary, in mice fed for over than 24 months with food contaminated by Malathion liver tumours were observed even at relatively low concentrations (USEPA, 2000b; National Pesticide Information Centre of USA). In addition, this compound is able to damage the nervous system of vertebrates through the inhibition of AChE (USEPA, 2000a); this effect causes the accumulation of ACh at the synapsis level: small excess of ACh causes over-stimulation of nervous system, while a great accumulation has the opposite effect (Gallo *et al.*, 1991).

The cholinergic system is a transmission system in which the molecules deputed to transfer the stimulation, such as ACh and other choline esters, work binding them to membrane receptors placed on the plasmalemma of target cells (Eusebi *et al.*, 1984).

ACh is a primary neurotransmitter of the sensory and neuromuscular system of several species and acts as a modulator of nerve impulse (Bozza Marrubini *et al.*, 1987; Ecobichon, 1991).

AChE is an enzyme occurring mainly in the nerve tissue and in muscles, it is located into the synapses between nerve and muscle cells and goes into action immediately after the passage of a signal; then ACh gives rise to acetic acid and choline, its two components; this mechanism holds the signal efficiently (Falugi & Raineri, 1985; Oettling *et al.*, 1985; Fluck, 1992). On the whole, AChE hydrolizes ACh and removes it fast from its receptor allowing the modulation of the signal (Lifshitz *et al.*, 1997).

Hence the inhibition of AChE leads to the accumulation of ACh that causes a permanent and excessive stimulation of nerve and muscle fibres: the postsynaptic membrane remains depolarized and the synaptic transmission does not occur (Forget & Bocquenè, 1999); this situation can lead to paralysis as well as to the organism death (Habig & Di Giulio, 1988; Galgani & Bocquenè, 1990; Payne *et al.*, 1996; Mc Henery *et al.*, 1997; Kirby *et al.*, 2000; Solè *et al.*, 2000; Forget *et al.*, 2003).

In this connection, the organophosphorus pesticides act on AChE blocking its catalytic site and preventing the ACh breaking by the enzyme (Bocquenè *et al.*, 1995; Forget & Bocquenè, 1999).

BIOMARKERS

A fundamental goal of ecotoxicological research concerns the evaluation of the effects consequent to the exposition of biota to pollutants. These responses are called 'biomarkers' and represent a signal of the environmental contamination; they are also indicators of the ecotoxic risk to which the natural populations are exposed (Bayne *et al.*, 1985; Mc Carthy & Shugart, 1990; Van der Oost *et al.*, 2003) and provide qualitative and semi-qualitative information about the damage and the relationships between the biological effects and the level of environmental contamination (Minutoli *et al.*, 2008).

In general, the early toxicity of a pollutant exerts at the biochemical and molecular level with modifications of enzyme activities, DNA alterations, etc., but subsequently through a cascade mechanism, the effects can be observed at the subsequent organization levels such as organelles, cell, tissue, whole organism, as far as to populations. The different homeostatic and non-homeostatic responses that the organism produces to counter the pollution are then potential biomarkers useful for the ecotoxicological assessment in the framework of environmental biomonitoring programmes (Mc Carthy & Shugart, 1990; Depledge, 1994). The assessment of the biomarkers in bioindicator organisms sampled in presumptively contaminated zones and in comparison with control organisms could allow to evaluate the potential risk of the whole concerned community (Depledge, 1989; Mc Carthy & Shugart, 1990; Fossi, 1991; Depledge, 1994).

Small crustaceans are an essential component of aquatic environments and a fundamental link in the food-web; for this reason, the evaluation of the ecotoxicological risk on these organisms through the biomarker approach can be an early signal of the ecosystem damage. As a matter of fact, to know the effects exerted on the lowest links of the food-web is useful to avoid the bioaccumulation and the biomagnification at the highest trophic levels (Minutoli *et al.*, 2008).

Tigriopus Fulvus as Target Organism

Copepods are often dominant among small crustaceans into the aquatic environments; for example, they represent the bulk of the planktonic biomass (Wells, 1984) and are the main connection between the phytoplankton and the higher trophic levels (Ruppert *et al.*, 2003).

These organisms occur in different habitats both as free forms and as parasites of teleosts and other organisms and can be also symbionts of several metazoans. Harpacticoid copepods play a very important role in the food-web being a food source for larval fish (Hicks & Coull, 1983); in addition, as from '70s of the last Century, some species have been adopted in ecotoxicological testing (D'Agostino & Finney, 1974; Bengtsson, 1978).

The genus *Tigriopus* spp. includes organisms that have been recently assumed a pre-eminent role in ecotoxicology and comprises the following species: *T. brevicornis* (Muller, 1776) typical of the Northern Atlantic coasts, *T. californicus* (Baker, 1912) typical of the Pacific coasts but sampled also in Eastern African coasts, *T. fulvus* (Fischer, 1860), living only in the Mediterranean splashpools, *T. japonicus* (Mori, 1938) that occurs in the Western Pacific coasts (Ito, 1970; Koga, 1970; Wells, 1976), *T. minutus* (Bozic, 1960) and *T. raki* (Bradford, 1967) typical of New Zealand splashpools, *T. brachydactilus* (Candeias, 1959) sampled along the coasts of Angola, *T. kerguelensis* (Soyer & Thiriot-Quevreux, 1985) found along the coasts of the Kerguelen Islands, *T. crozettensis* (Soyer & Thiriot-Quevreux, 1985) found along the coasts of the Crozet Islands, *T. angulatus* (Lang, 1933) observed along the coasts of the Macquarie, Campbell and Tasmania Islands.

Tigripous fulvus is an autochtonous harpacticoid of the Mediterranean coasts, living in the supralittoral splashpools of the rocky shores characterized by wide fluctuations of the environmental conditions (Carli & Fiori, 1977; Pane *et al.*, 2001; Pane & Mariottini, 2010). It has small size, lengthened and cylindrical body and it is red-orange coloured due to the astaxanthin pigment; the length of females ranges between 0.7 and 0.75 mm, while the males are a little longer (0.8 – 0.85 mm). A remarkable sexual dimorphism allows to recognize easily the sex. *T. fulvus* feeds mainly on bacteria, diatoms such as *Thalassiosira* sp. and microalgae such as *Tetraselmis* spp. (Powlik *et al.*, 1997): the food is directed to the mouth and is filtered by mouthparts.

The life cycle of *T. fulvus* extends over 75 days on average with maximum of around 100 days; the reproductive period of the female extends over 49 days on the average with maximum of over 80 days (Carli *et al.*, 1989a).

T. fulvus reproduces all year round but mainly from spring to autumn. Females are very fertile and after an unique mating they produce on the average ten egg-sacs (Carli *et al.*, 1989a) containing agglutinated eggs (Fraser, 1936). The first egg-sac is given out 7-10 days after mating; after hatching of an egg-sac the subsequent one appears two days later on the average (Carli *et al.*, 1989a).

The egg sacs, at first dark green-coloured, grow fast assuming a pale green and then a bright orange colour. In the last phase small red spots are visible revealing the development of the ocular pigment of embryos.

The population structure of *T. fulvus* seems to be affected by seasonal variations of water temperature and of suspended particulate matter. Population density is characterized by an annual trend and copepodites and adults show different abundance peaks (Pane *et al.*, 1996).

In ecotoxicological testing is essential to have at disposal test-species that are: I) easily found in the natural environment, II) easily breeded in the laboratory, III) sensitive to diverse xenobiotics; furthermore experimental methods applicable to the diverse environmental matrices are needing. In this connection, copepods are used especially because they play an important role owing to their key-position in the aquatic food-web. In particular *Tigriopus fulvus*, whose the life-cycle (Carli *et al.*, 1989a, 1995), ecology (Pane *et al.*, 1996), energetic content (Pane *et al.*, 2003), fatty acid composition (Carli *et al.*, 1989b) and the association with adhering vibrios (Carli *et al.*, 1993; Pane *et al.*, 2000) are well-known, is for long the object of ecotoxicological studies (Todaro *et al.*, 2001; Faraponova *et al.*, 2005; Pane *et al.*, 2005; Pane *et al.*, 2008) and was indicated as eligible to the role of test-species to define standardized methods (Pane *et al.*, 2007) thanks to its constant availability in splashpools (Pane *et al.*, 1996; Pane and Mariottini, 2010), easy breeding and high fertility (Carli *et al.*, 1989a), small size (Fraser, 1936; Harris, 1973; Wells, 1976) and low costs to carry out the tests. Furthermore, a fundamental aspect concerns the possibility to obtain enough numerous and homogeneous cohorts through the stimulation of hatching of mature eggs, recognizable for the colour as well as for the evidence of the embryo naupliar eye (Pane *et al.*, 2005).

Materials and Methods

The tests were carried out exposing *T. fulvus* ovigerous females to the organophosphorus pesticide Malathion; treated organisms were then used to evaluate the biomarkers related to the enzyme activity of AChE.

The specimens were sampled in a supralittoral coastal rocky shore of the Ligurian Sea (Genova-Nervi), acclimatized in the laboratory in Instant Ocean® artificial seawater filtered with 0.45 μm filters, at salinity 37 PSU, temperature 20±0.5 °C, light:dark cycle 16:8 hours and fed *ad libitum* with commercial food (Salt Creek Feeds for Aquaculture, Salt Lake City, USA), unicellular algae *Tetraselmis suecica* and commercial yeast *Saccharomyces cerevisiae*.

In order to obtain same-aged nauplii to be used after reaching of adult stage in toxicity tests, 100-200 ovigerous females were collected from the laboratory culture and egg hatching was stimulated by gentle detaching of mature egg sacs with fine needles after immobilization of females on Whatman GF/F filters, leaving a thin water layer to avoid any damage (Pane *et al.*, 2005). After reaching of adult stage and after emission of the first egg-sac same-aged females were put in multiwell plates and the tests were carried out in triplicate on 10 copepods per well with scalar dilutions of the pesticide. Two untreated controls (each in triplicate) were prepared the first with Instant Ocean® seawater and the second with a solution of 0.1% acetone in seawater, equivalent to the solvent concentration of the highest Malathion concentration (800 μg/l). In the tests an appropriate amount of specimens (90 per concentration) were utilized modifying what suggested by Forget *et al.* (2003) and Cailleaud *et al.* (2007).

The stock solution (1 g/l) was prepared dissolving Malathion in acetone 100%; the following dilutions in Instant Ocean® artificial seawater, chosen after preliminary tests, were used: 1.56 μg/l, 3.12 μg/l, 6.25 μg/l, 12.5 μg/l, 25 μg/l, 50 μg/l, 100 μg/l, 200 μg/l, 400 μg/l and 800 μg/l. The tests were carried out at 20 °C; during the test the organisms were not fed.

After 24, 48 and 96 hours of treatment dead organisms were counted; when possible the No Observed Effect Concentration (NOEC) of the activity of the studied enzyme was determined. Then all specimens were collected and frozed at -20 °C until the biomarker analysis. Dead organisms were not considered in the analyses owing to the fast denaturation of proteins; for this reason, the biomarker evaluation was performed only with a mortality lower than 10%.

Homogenates were obtained according to Forget *et al.*, 2003 modified and to Cailleaud *et al.*, 2007 modified, with a Polytron PT 300 (Kinematica) homogenizer from 90 ovigerous females (around 90 mg wet weight) per tested concentration suspending them in 270 μl of Na-phosphate 0.01 M buffer with 0.1% Triton X-100 at pH 7 (1:4 weight/volume). Then the homogenates were centrifuged (BR 4i, Jouan; 15 minutes at 2,000 rpm, 4 °C) to remove the large particulate and the supernatant was re-centrifuged (4 °C, 30 minutes, 12,000 rpm). Finally the supernatant was collected and frozen at -20 °C until analysis.

The AChE activity was evaluated according to the colorimetric method of Ellman *et al.* (1960) with modifications, using Acetyl-β-(methyl)thiocoline iodide (AcTChI) as substrate and Ditio-bis-nitrobenzoate (DTNB) as reagent.

The quantitative determination of total proteins was performed according to Bradford (1976). The samples were analyzed in triplicate; the absorbance value was converted into μg of total proteins per μl of homogenate. Analytical grade reagents were used (Sigma-Aldrich, Milano; Fluka, Milano; Bio-Rad Laboratories, Segrate - Milano).

RESULTS

After 24 and 48 hours of treatment mortality was not observed, or it was very low, at all concentrations; on the contrary, after 96 hours was not possible to carry out the enzyme analysis for the concentrations 200, 400 and 800 μg/l that caused higher than 10% mortality.

The values of AChE activity in the samples treated with Malathion for 24, 48 and 96 hours are shown in tab. 1.

After 24 hours enzyme inhibition increased with increasing of Malathion concentration. It should be considered that only ≥20% inhibition compared to the control are indicated to be significant (USEPA, 1998), thus the Lowest Observed Effect Concentration (LOEC) was 25 μg/l and consequently the (NOEC) was 12.5 μg/l.

After 48 hours a similar trend was observed, but after a sharp initial drop the inhibition carried on more gradually. As expected, NOEC e LOEC values decreased and the lowest tested concentration (1.56 μg/l) caused > 20% inhibition.

After 96 hours of treatment the lowest concentrations showed AChE activity comparable to controls only from 12.5 μg/l (LOEC) onwards the AChE inhibition resulted significant.

The specific activity of AChE as percent inhibition in comparison with the control (0.1% acetone in artificial seawater) after 24, 48 and 96 ore of treatment with Malathion is shown in Figure 1.

Table 1. AChE activity after 24, 48 and 96 hours of treatment with Malathion. Ctrl = control with artificial seawater; ctr2 = control with 0.1% acetone in seawater

tested concentrations (μg/l)	time		
	24 hours	48 hours	96 hours
	nmol/mg total proteins/minute		
ctr 1	181	300	85
ctr 2	127	197	107
1.56	123	154	87
3.12	116	136	91
6.25	109	76	101
12.5	111	121	57
25	95	143	67
50	87	70	53
100	97	92	48
200	65	96	-
400	95	40	-
800	73	70	-

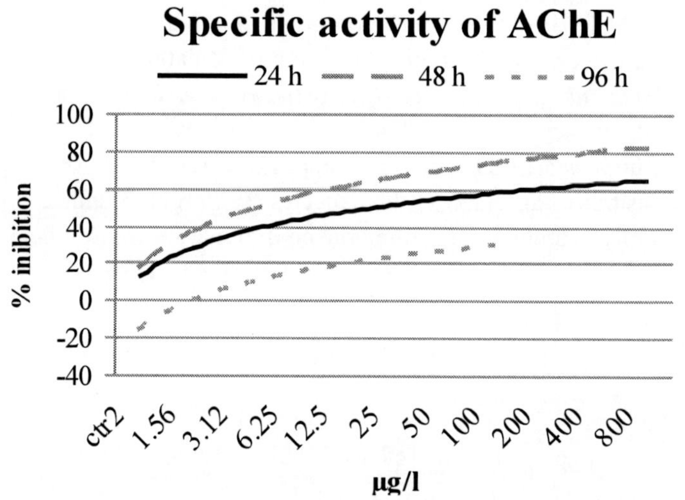

Figure 1. AChE specific activity as percent inhibition in comparison with ctr2 (control with 0.1% acetone in artificial seawater) after 24, 48 and 96 ore of treatment with Malathion.

CONCLUSION

AChE analysis showed that enzyme activity decreases when pesticide concentration increases in all treatments (24, 48 and 96 hours). Considering that only 20% inhibition indicates a manifest toxic effect (USEPA, 1998), after 24 hours of treatment a significant inhibition was obtained from 25 μg/l onwards; otherwise, after 48 hours the inhibition was more pronounced and evident starting from lower concentrations. After 96 hours the lower tested concentrations showed a non-significant inhibition and only from 12.5 μg/l (LOEC) started the decrease of enzyme activity that nevertheless did not reach the results observed after 48 hours. These observations could be the result of a tolerance after prolonged exposition to a determined substance, a phenomenon already known in the pharmacological research (Romero et al., 1998; Donckier et al., 2006; Bourova et al., 2010) and observed during *in vitro* experiments (Martin & Garcia de Jalon, 1982).

Tests on AChE activity in the hemolimph of *Carcinus maenas* exposed to Dimethoate have shown that significant effects were observed as from treatments with 2 mg/l with enzyme activity that passing from 254±109 nmol/mg total proteins/minute before treatment to 194±91 nmol/mg total proteins/minute after 24 hours treatment (Lundebye *et al.*, 1997); whereas our results show the occurrence of significant effects as from lower concentration (25 μg/l).

In the freshwater crustacean *Gammarus pulex* the AChE inhibition caused by Chlorpyriphos was 50% after 96 hours of treatment with 0.35 (0.32-0.36) μg/l (Xuereb *et al.*, 2007). AChE inhibition tests in *Daphnia magna* showed the EC_{50}s 48 hours were 2.4 μg/l and 0.2 μg/l after treatment with Parathion and with Paraoxon respectively (Guilhermino *et al.*, 1996).

Malathion induces AChE inhibition also on mammals: oral administration of 100, 500 and 1500 ppm for 4 weeks were seen to inhibit respectively 45, 48 and 51% AChE in plasma and 73, 75 and 78% AChE in slaver of rats (Abdollahi *et al.*, 2004).

In conclusion, this work demonstrates the action of Malathion on AChE activity and the suitability of *Tigriopus fulvus* as a model to study the ecotoxicity of pesticides mainly for the characteristics of its life-cycle, as well as for its easy availability and breeding in the laboratory, for its high sensitivity and for the positive responses to the performed tests. Therefore, the possibility to employ this species as target-organism in environmental monitoring, and mainly in studies concerning the coastal marine environment, is confirmed.

REFERENCES

Abdollahi, M., Ranjbar, A., Shadnia, S., Nikfar, S. & Rezaie, A. (2004). *Pesticides and oxidative stress: a review.* Medical Science Monitor, **10**, RA 141-147.

Aluigi, M. G., Angelini, C., Corte, G. & Falugi C. (2008). *The sea urchin, Paracentrotus lividus, embryo as a "bioethical" model for neurodevelopmental toxicity testing: effects of diazinon on the intracellular distribution of OTX2-like proteins.* Cell Biology and Toxicology, 24 (6), 587-601.

ARPAL (2004). *Monitoraggio dei sedimenti e delle biocenosi marine. Raccolta, adeguamento ed integrazione delle informazioni.* CTN-AIM.

Bacci, E. (1994). *Ecotoxicology of Organic Contaminants.* Boca Raton, FL, USA, Lewis Publishers.

Baker, B. (1912). *Notes on the Crustacea of Laguna Beach.* First annual report of the Laguna Marine Laboratory at Laguna Beach, Orange County, California, USA, 110

Bayne, B. L., Brown, D. A., Burns, K., Dixon, D. R., Ivanovici, A., Livingstone, D. R., Lowe, D. M., Moore, M. N., Stebbing, A. R. D. & Widdows, J. (1985). *The effects of stress and pollution on marine animals.* New York, USA, Prager Scientific.

Bengtsson, B. E. (1978). *Use of a harpacticoid copepod in toxicity tests*. Marine Pollution Bulletin, 9, 238-241.

Bocquenè, G., Bellanger, C. & Cadiou, Y. (1995). *Joint action of combinations of pollutants in the acetylcholinesterase activity of several marine species*. Ecotoxicology, 4, 266-279.

Bourova, L., Vosahlikova, M., Kagan, D., Dlouha, K., Novotny, J. & Svoboda, P. (2010). *Long-term adaptation to high doses of morphine causes desensitization of mu-OR- and delta-OR-stimulated G-protein response in forebrain cortex but does not decrease the amount of G-protein alpha subunits*. Medical Science Monitor, 16 (8), BR260-270.

Bozic, B. (1960). *Le genre Tigriopus (Norman) (Copépodes, Harpacticoides) et ses formes Européennes*. Reserches morphologiques et expérimentales. Archives of Zoological Experimental Genetics, 93, 169-269.

Bozza Marrubini, M., Ghezzi Laurenzi, R. & Uccelli, P. (1987). *Intossicazioni acute: meccanismi, diagnosi e terapia.* 2ª edizione. Milano, Italy, Organizzazione Editoriale Medico Farmaceutica (OEMF).

Bradford, J. M. (1967). *The genus Tigriopus (Norman) (Copepoda, Harpacticoida) in New Zealand with a description of a new species.* Transactions of the Royal Society of New Zealand, Zoology, 10, 51-59.

Bradford, M. M. (1976). *A rapid and sensitive method for the quantitation of microgram quantities of protein utilizing the principle of protein-dye binding.* Analytical Biochemistry, 72, 248-254.

Brodie, J. E. & Mitchell, A. V. (2005). *Nutrients in Australian tropical rivers: changes with agricultural development and implications for receiving environments.* Marine and Freshwater Research, 56, 279-302.

Cailleaud, K., Maillet, G., Budzinski, H., Souissi, S. & Forget-Leray, J. (2007). *Effects of salinity on the expression of enzymatic biomarkers in Eurytemora affinis (Calanoida, Copepoda).* Comparative Biochemistry and Physiology, Part A Molecular Integrative Physiology, 147 (4), 841-849.

Candeias, A. (1959). *Contribution to the knowledge of the Harpacticoids (Crustacea, Copepoda) from the littoral of Angola*. Publicações Culturais da Companhia de Diamantes de Angola, Portugal, 45, 79-104.

Carli, A. & Fiori, M. A. (1977). *Sullo sviluppo larvale del Tigriopus fulvus (Fischer).* Atti IX Congresso S.I.B.M.; Lacco Ameno d'Ischia 19-22 Maggio 1977, 181-190.

Carli, A., Mariottini, G. L. & Pane, L. (1989a). *Reproduction of the rockpools harpacticoid copepod Tigriopus fulvus, suitable for aquaculture*. Bulletin de l'Institut Océanographique de Monaco, spec. 5, 295-300.

Carli, A., Balestra, V., Pane, L. & Valente, T. (1989b). *Rapporto di composizione percentuale degli acidi grassi nel Tigriopus fulvus delle pozze di scogliera della costa ligure.* Bollettino della Società Italiana di Biologia Sperimentale, 55, 421-427.

Carli, A., Pane, L., Casareto, L., Bertone, S. & Pruzzo, C. (1993). *Occurrence of Vibrio alginolyticus in Ligurian coast rock pools (Tyrrhenian Sea, Italy) and its association with the copepod Tigriopus fulvus (Fischer, 1860).* Applied Environmental Microbiology, 59, 1960-1962.

Carli,A., Mariottini, G. L. & Pane, L. (1995). *Influence of nutrition on fecundity and survival in Tigriopus fulvus Fischer (Copepoda, Harpacticoida).* Aquaculture, 134, 113-119.

Carli, A., Pane, L. & Mariottini, G. L. (1998). *Elementi di Ecologia Applicata. n. 6, Ecotossicologia.* Genova, Italy, ECIG Edizioni.

Christensen, B. T., Lauridsen, T. L., Ravn, H. W. & Bayley, M. (2005). *A comparison of feeding efficiency and swimming ability of Daphnia magna exposed to cypermethrin.* Aquatic Toxicology, 73, 210-220.

Dagnino, A., Allen, J. I., Moore, M. N., Broeg, K., Canesi, L. & Viarengo, A. (2007). *Development of an expert system for the integration of biomarker responses in mussels into an animal health index.* Biomarkers, 12 (2), 155-172.

D'Agostino, A. & Finney, C. (1974). *The effect of copper and cadmium on the development of Tigriopus japonicus.* In: Vemberg, W. B., editor. Pollution and Physiology of Marine Organisms. New York, USA, Academic Press; 445-463.

Dahr, G., Barat, S. & Dahr, K. M. (2004). *Influence of the organophosphorus insecticide phosphamidon on lentic water.* Journal of Environmental Biology, 25, 359-363.

Depledge, M. H. (1989). *The rational basis for detection of the early effects of marine pollutants using physiological indicators.* AMBIO, 18, 301-302.

Depledge, M. H. (1994). *The rational basis for the use of biomarkers as ecotoxicological tools.* In: Fossi, M. C., Leonzio, C., editors. Nondestructive Biomarkers in Vertebrates. Boca Raton, FL, USA, Lewis Publishers; 261-285.

Donckier, V., Troisi, R., Le Moine, A., Toungouz, M., Ricciardi, S., Colle, I., Van Vlierberghe, H., Craciun, L., Libin, M., Praet, M., Noens, L., Stordeur, P., Andrien, M., Lambermont, M., Gelin, M., Bourgeois, N., Adler, M., de Hemptinne, B. & Goldman, M. (2006). *Early immunosuppression withdrawal after living donor liver transplantation and donor stem cell infusion.* Liver Transplantation, 12, 1523-1528.

Duursma, E. K. & Marchard, M. (1974). *Aspect of organic marine pollution.* Oceanography and Marine Biology: Annual Review, 12, 315-431.

Ecobichon, D. J. (1991). *Toxic effects of pesticides.* In: Amdur, M. O., Doull, J. & Klaassen, C. D., editors. Casarett and Doull's Toxicology. New York, USA, Pergamon, 565-622.

Ellman, G. L., Courtney, K. D., Andres, V. & Featherstone, R. M. (1960). *A new rapid colorimetric determination of Acetylcholinesterase activity.* Biochemical Pharmacology, 7, 88-95.

EPA (2002). *Methods for measuring the acute toxicity of effluents and receiving waters to freshwater and marine organisms.* Fifth Edition. October 2002. EPA-821-R-02-012.

Eusebi, F., Pasetto, N. & Siracusa, G. (1984). *Acethylcholine receptors in human oocytes.* Journal of Physiology, 346, 321-330.

Falugi, C & Raineri, M. (1985). *Acetylcholinesterase and pseudocholinesterase activity distribution pattern in early developing chick limbs.* Journal of Embryology and Experimental Morphology, 86, 89-108.

Faraponova, O., De Pascale, D., Onorati, F. & Finoia, M. G. (2005). *Tigriopus fulvus (Copepoda, Harpacticoida) as a target species in biological assays.* Meiofauna Marina, 14, 91-95.

Fischer, S. (1860). *Beitrage zur Kenntniss der Entomostraca.* Abhandlungen der Baierischen Akademie der Wissenschaften, 8, 656-660.

Fleeger, J. W., Carman, K.R. & Nisbet, R. M. (2003). *Indirect effects of contaminants in aquatic ecosystems.* Science of the Total Environment, 317, 207-233.

Fluck, R. A. (1992). *Localization of acetylcholinesterase activity in young embryos of the medaka Oryzias latipes, a teleost.* Comparative Biochemistry and Physiology C, 72(1), 59-64.

Forget, J., Beliaeff, B. & Bocquenè, G. (2003). *Acetylcholinesterase activity in copepods (Tigriopus brevicornis) from the Vilaine River estuary, France, as a biomarker of neurotoxic contaminants.* Aquatic Toxicology, 62, 195-204.

Forget, J. & Bocquenè, G. (1999). *Partial purification and enzymatic characterization of acetylcholinesterase from the intertidal marine copepod Tigriopus brevicornis.* Comparative Biochemistry and Physiology B, 123, 345-350.

Fossi, M. C. (1991). *L'utilizzo dei biomarkers nella valutazione del rischio ambientale: metodologie ed applicazione.* Inquinamento, 12, 44-50.

Fraser, J. H. (1936). *The occurrence, ecology and life history of Tigriopus fulvus (Fischer).* Journal of the Marine Biological Association of the United Kingdom, 20, 253-536.

Galgani, F. & Bocquenè, G. (1990). *In vitro inhibition of acetylcholinesterase from four marine species by organophosphates and carbamates.* Bulletin of Environmental Contamination and Toxicology, 45, 243-249.

Gallo, M. A. & Lawryk, N. J. (1991). *Organic Phosphorus Pesticides.* In: Hayes, W. J., Laws, E. R., editors. Handbook of Pesticide Toxicology. San Diego, CA, USA, Academic Press; 2, 917-112

Guilhermino, L., Lopes, M. C., Carvalho, A. P. & Soares, A. M. V. M. (1996). *Inhibition of acetylcholinesterase activity as effect criterion in acute tests with juvenile Daphnia magna.* Chemosphere, 32 (4), 721-738.

Habig, C. & Di Giulio, R. T. (1988). *The anticholinesterase effects of the cotton defoliant S,S,S,-tri-n-butyl phosphorotrithioate (DEF) on channel catfish.* Marine Environmental Research, 24, 193-197.

Harris, R. P. (1973). *Feeding, growth, reproduction and nitrogen utilization by the harpacticoid copepod Tigriopus brevicornis.* Journal of the Marine Biological Association of the United Kingdom, 54, 141-155.

Hazardous Substances Data Bank (HSDB) (2000) [CD-ROM]; U.S. *National Library of Medicine:* Bethesda, MD, USA. Malathion.

Hicks, G. R. F. & Coull, B. C. (1983). *The ecology of marine meiobenthic harpacticoid copepods.* Oceanography and Marine Biology: Annual Review, 21, 380-389.

Hornsby, A. G., Wauchope, D. R. & Herner, A. E. (1999). *Pesticide Properties in the Environment;* New York, USA, Springer.

Howard, P. H. (1991). *Handbook of Environmental Fate and Exposure Date for Organic Chemicals.* Chelsea, MI, USA, Lewis.

Islam, M. S. & Tanaka, M. (2004). *Impacts of pollution on coastal and marine ecosystem including coastal and marine fisheries and approach for management: a review and synthesis.* Marine Pollution Bulletin, 48, 624-649.

Ito, T. (1970). *The biology of a harpacticoid copepod, Tigriopus japonicus Mori.* Journal of the Faculty of Sciences. Hokkaido University, Ser. VI, Zoology, 17, 474-499.

Jamal, G. A., Hansen, S. & Julu, P. O. (2002). *Low level exposures to organophosphorus esters may cause neurotoxicity.* Toxicology, 181-182: 23-33.

James, C. S., Fisher, J., Russell, V., Collings, S. & Moss, B. (2005). *Nitrate availability and hydrophyte species richness in shallow lakes.* Freshwater Biology, 50, 1049-1063.

Karczmar, A. G., Ishi, S. & Blaber, L. C. (1970). *Investigations, particularly by means of the anticholinesterase agents, of the multiple peripheral and central cholinergic mechanisms and of their behavioural implications.* Acta Vitaminologica et Enzymologica, 24(4), 131-189.

Kirby, M. F., Morris, S., Hurst, M., Kirby, S. J., Neall, P., Tylor, T. & Fagg, A. (2000). *The use of cholinesterase activity in flounder (Platichthys flesus) muscle tissue as a biomarker of neurotoxic contamination in UK estuaries.* Marine Pollution Bulletin, 40, 780-791.

Koga, F. (1970). *On the life history of Tigriopus japonicus Mori (Copepoda).* Journal of the Oceanographic Society of Japan, 26, 12-21.

Lang, K. (1933). *Zwei neue Brackwasserharpacticieden von den Macquarie Inseln.* K. fysiogr. Sallsk. I Lund Forh, 3, 1-14.

Lifshitz, M., Shahak, E. & Bolotin, A. (1997). *Carbamate poisoning in early childhood and in adults.* Clinical Toxicology, 35, 25-27.

Lundebye, A. K., Curtis, T. M., Braven, J. & Depledge, M. H. (1997). *Effects of the organophosphorous pesticide, dimethoate, on cardiac and acetylcholinesterase (AChE) activity in the shore crab Curcinus maenas.* Aquatic Toxicology, 40, 23-36.

Marchetti, R. (1993). *Ecologia applicata.* Società Italiana di Ecologia. Milano, Italy, Città Studi.

Marrs, T. C. (1997). *Malathion. In: Pesticide residues in food, Joint FAO/WHO Meeting on Pesticide Residues, Evaluations: Part II – Toxicol. Environ. Chem.*; International Programme on Chemical Safety. World Health Organization: Geneva, Switzerland; 189-219.

Martin, I. A. A. & Garcia de Jalon, P. (1982). *Sensitization by in vitro incubation with morphine of the myenteric plexus-longitudinal muscle preparation.* Journal of Pharmacology, 13 (1), 3-10.

Mc Carthy, F. & Shugart, L.R. (1990). *Biomarkers of environmental contamination.* Chelsea, USA, Lewis Publisher.

Mc Henery, J. G., Linley-Adams, G. E., Moore, D. C., Rodger, G. K. & Davies, I. M. (1997). *Experimental field studies of effects of dichlorvos exposure on acetylcholinesterase activity in the gill of the mussel, Mytilus edulis L.* Aquatic Toxicology, 38, 125-143.

Minutoli, R., Fossi, M. C., Zagami, G., Granata, A. & Guglielmo, L. (2008). *First application of biomarkers approach in the zooplanktonic copepod Acartia latisetosa for the early management and conservation of transitional waters ecosystems.* Transitional Waters Bulletin, 1, 45-52.

Mori, T. (1938). *Tigriopus japonicus, a new species of a neritic Copepoda.* Zoological Magazine, 50 (5), 249-295.

Moss, B. (2001). *Continental-scale patterns of nutrient and fish effects on shallow lakes: synthesis of a pan-European mesocosms experiment.* Freshwater Biology, 49, 1633-1649.

Moss, B. (2008). *Water pollution by agriculture.* Philosophical Transactions of the Royal Society B: Biological Sciences, 363, 659-666.

Muller. O. F. (1776). *Zoologiae Danicae Prodromus: seu animalium Daniae et Norvegiae indigenarum characteres, nomina, et synonyma imprimis popularium.* Havniae (Copenhagen), 1-292.

NPIC-*National Pesticide Information Centre.* http://npic.orst.edu/

NRC (1989). *Biologic markers in reproductive toxicology.* Washington, D.C., USA, National Academy Press.

Oddo, N. (2001). *Ecotossicologia: definizione, campo di applicazione, obiettivi.* Biologi Italiani, 8, 54-57.

Oettling, G., Schmidt, H. & Drews, U. (1985). *The muscarinic receptor of chick embryos cells: correlation between ligand binding and calcium mobilization.* Journal of Cell Biology, 100(4), 1073-1081.

Olson, B. M., Miller, J. J., Rodvang, S. J. & Yanke, J. L. (2005). *Soil and groundwater quality under a cattle feedlot in southern Alberta.* Water Quality Research Foundation, Canada, 40, 131-144.

Pane, L., Feletti, M. & Carli, A. M. (1996). *Fattori ambientali e fluttuazioni della popolazione del copepode Tigriopus fulvus delle pozze di scogliera di Genova-Nervi.* S. It. E. Atti, 17, 317-320.

Pane, L., De Nuccio, L., Pruzzo, C. & Carli, A. (2000). *Adhesion of bacteria and diatoms to the exoskeleton of the harpacticoid copepod Tigriopus fulvus in culture: electron and epifluorescent microscope study.* Journal of Biological Research – Bollettino della Società Italiana di Biologia Sperimentale, 76, 37-43.

Pane, L., Capelli, R., Paganelli, L. & Carli, A. M. (2001). *Inorganic mercury in the rock pool environment (Ligurian Sea).* Journal of Biological Research – Bollettino della Società Italiana di Biologia Sperimentale, 77 (1-3), 7-12.

Pane, L., De Nuccio, L. & Franceschi, E. (2003). *Energy value of the copepod Tigriopus fulvus (Fischer, 1860): application of DSC technique (Differential Scanning Calorimetry).* Biologia Marina Mediterranea, 10 (2), 593-596.

Pane, L., Giacco, E. & Mariottini, G. L. (2005). *Acute and chronic heavy metal biomass on Tigriopus fulvus (Fischer) (Copepoda: Harpacticoida).* 13th Symp. PRIMO 13, Alessandria, Italy, June 19-22. Book of abstracts, 13

Pane, L., Giacco, E. & Mariottini, G. L. (2007). *Effect of surfactants on the reproduction of Tigriopus fulvus Fischer.* Experimental Biology Reports, 1 (1), 1-12.

Pane, L., Mariottini, G. L., Lodi, A. & Giacco E. (2008). *Effects of heavy metals on laboratory reared Tigriopus fulvus Fischer (Copepoda Harpacticoida).* In: Brown, S. E., Welton, W. C., editors, Heavy Metal Pollution. Hauppauge, NY, Nova Science Publishers Inc.; Chapter 6, 157-165.

Pane, L. & Mariottini G.L. 2010. *Characteristics of the rocky littoral system. Biological and ecological aspects.* In: Macias, B., Guajardo, F. editors, Rock Chemistry. Hauppauge, NY., Nova Science Publishers, Inc.; Chapter 5, 121-130.

Payne, J., Mathieu, A., Melvin, W. & Fancey L.L. (1996). *Acetylcholinesterase, an old biomarker with a new future? Field trials in association with two urban rivers and a paper mill in Newfoundland.* Marine Pollution Bulletin, 32, 225-231.

Powe, M., Attrill, M. J. & Thomas, R. M. (1999). *Trends in agricultural pesticide (atrazine, lindane, simazine) concentration in the Thames estuary.* Environmental Pollution., 104, 31-39.

Powlik, J. J., Lewis, A. G. & Spaeth, M. (1997). *Development, body length, and feeding of Tigriopus californicus (Copepoda Harpacticoida) in laboratory and field populations.* Crustaceana, 70, 324-343.

Pretty, J. N., Mason, C. F., Nedwell, D. B. & Hine, R. E. (2003). *Environmental costs of freshwater eutrophication in England and Wales.* Environmental Science and Technology, 37, 201-208.

Raven, P. J., Holmes, N. T. H., Dawson, F. H., Fox, P. J. A., Everard, M., Fozzard, I. R. & Rowen, K. J. (1998). *River habitat quality. River habitat survey report.* Environment Agency, Bristol, UK.

Romero, J. N., Berrendero, F., Manzanares, J., Pérez, A., Corchero, J., Fuentes, J. A., Fernández-Ruiz, J. J. & Ramos, J. A. (1998). *Time-coursc of the cannabinoid receptor down-regulation in the adult rat brain caused by repeated exposure to D9-Tetrahydrocannabinol.* Synapse, 30, 298-308.

Ruppert, E. E., Fox, R. S. & Barnes, R. D. (2003). *Invertebrate Zoology. A Functional Evolutionary Approach,* 7th ed., Belmont, CA, USA. Brooks/Cole-Thomson Learning,

Solè, M., Porte, C., Barcelo, D. & Albaiges, G. (2000). *Bivalves residue analysis for assessment of coastal pollution in the Ebro delta (NW Mediterranean Sea).* Marine Pollution Bulletin, 40, 746-753.

Soyer, J. & Thiriot-Quievreux, C. (1985). *Existence d'espéces jumelle dans le genre Tigriopus (Copepoda, Harpacticoida) aux Iles Kerguelen et Crozet (Terres Australes et Antarctique Françaises).* Comptes Rendus de l'Académie des Sciences, Paris, 301(III), 309-312.

Sultatos, L. G. (1994). *Mammalian toxicology of organophosphorus pesticides.* Journal of Toxicology and Environmental Health, 43(3), 271-289.

Thiere, G. & Shulz R. (2004). *Runoff-related agricultural impact in relation to macroinvertebrate communities of the Lourens River*, South Africa. Water Research, 38, 3092-3102.

Todaro, M. A., Faraponova, O., Onorati, F., Pellegrini, D. & Tongiorgi, P. (2001). *Tigriopus fulvus (Copepoda, Harpacticoida) a possible test-species in harbour sediment toxicity bioassessment: life cycle and preliminary bioassays.* Biologia Marina Mediterranea, 8 (1), 869-872.

Traas, T. P., Jansen, J. H., Van den Brink, P. J., Brock, T. C. M. & Aldenberg, T. (2004). *A freshwater food web model for the combined effects of nutrients and insecticide stress and subsequent recovery.* Environmental Toxicology and Chemistry, 23, 521-529.

US EPA, (1988). *Office of Pesticide Programs*, U.S. Government Printing Office: Washington, DC. Pesticide Fact Sheet Number 152: Malathion.

US EPA (1998). *Science Policy Issues Related to the Food Quality Protection Act. Office of pesticide program's science policy on the use of cholinesterase inhibition for the risk assessment of organophosphate and carbamate pesticides, OPP Docket #00560, Federal Register 63.* US Environmental Protection Agency, 214.

US EPA, (2000a). *Office of Pesticide Programs*, Washington, DC. Malathion Preliminary Risk Assessments: Environmental Fate and Effects. www.epa.gov.

US EPA, (2000b). *Office of Pesticide Programs*, Washington, DC. Malathion Preliminary Risk Assessments: Toxicology Chapter. www.epa.gov.

Van der Oost, R., Beyer, J. & Vermeulen, N. P. E. (2003). *Fish bioaccumulation and biomarkers in environmental risk assessment: a review.* Environmental Toxicology and Pharmacology, 13, 57-149.

Vighi, M. (1989). *Ecotossicologia. Guida Generale Organica sull'Ambiente.* Milano, Italy, Edizioni Giuridico-Scientifiche.

Vismara, R. (1992). *Ecologia Applicata. Inquinamento e salute umana, criteri di protezione dell'aria, delle acque, del suolo, valutazione di impatto ambientale, esempi di calcolo.* Milano, Italy, Ulrico Hoepli Editore.

Wells, J. B. J. (1976). *Keys to Aid in the Identification of Marine Harpacticoid Copepods.* Aberdeen, UK, The Aberdeen University Press Ltd.

Wells, P. G. (1984). *Marine ecotoxicological tests with zooplankton.* In: Persoone, G., Jaspers, E., Claus, C., editors. Ecotoxicological Testing for the Marine Enviroment, vol. 1. Bredene, Belgium, Institute for Marine Scientific Research, 215-256.

Widdows, J. (1994*). Handbook of Ecotoxicology.* In: Calow P. editor. Marine and Estuarine Toxicity Tests. Sheffield, UK, Department of Animal and Plant Sciences, University of Sheffield; 145-146

Williams, W. D. & Aladin, N. V. (1991). *The Aral Sea: recent limnological changes in their conservation significance.* Aquatic Conservation: Marine and Freshwater Ecosystems, 1, 3-24.

Xuereb, B., Noury, P., Felten, V., Garric, J. & Geffard, O. (2007). *Cholinesterase activity in Gammarus pulex (Crustacea Amphipoda): Characterization and effects of chlorpyrifos.* Toxicology, 236, 178–189.

In: Xenobiotics: New Research
Editors: Saul F. Castaneda and Mauro L. Emerson
ISBN: 978-1-61942-616-0

Chapter 4

TRANSFORMATION OF HERBICIDES UNDER TRANSIENT ANOXIA

Gerald K. Sims[1] and Ramdas Gopinath Kanissery[2]
[1]Agricultural Research Service, United States Department of Agriculture
[2]Department of Natural Resources and Environmental Sciences,
University of Illinois, 1102 South Goodwin Avenue, Urbana, IL, US

ABSTRACT

Resurgence in the use of soil-applied residual herbicides to augment performance of failing post-emergence herbicides has predictably reignited concerns over potential offsite movement, carryover damage onsite, or potential herbicide failure due to accelerated degradation. Many of the key processes in herbicide fate are relatively well-described, however, the bulk of our knowledge of herbicide transformation in soil is based on assumed aerobic conditions, which leaves gaps in our understanding of events taking place during transient saturation. Many areas of agricultural production are vulnerable to periodic flooding, which results in slower O_2 replenishment, and thus promotes local anoxia. Variation in water content through its extremes modulates the bioavailability of substrates to microorganisms, as well as the dominant types of organisms and their associated activities (due to fluctuation of redox regime). Most information about anaerobic processes of herbicide degradation in soil has been derived from experiments performed under long-term submersion, however some studies have demonstrated significant impact of even transient soil saturation on herbicide degradation. A thorough analysis of available data is needed not only to address the current frequency of soil saturation events, but also anticipated changes in water regime as global climates shift. For example, in the American Midwest, projected changes in rainfall patterns are expected to have profound influence on soil water status and variability. Herein, we review literature available on herbicide fate processes as a function of soil water regime, including transient flooding. Examples are presented of herbicides undergoing degradation under denitrifying and iron-reducing conditions, which are most likely to be encountered under transient flooding. New findings are presented for reductive dehalogenation and potential for this process under transient flooding. Also described are water effects on the ecology and activities of herbicide-degrading microorganisms, as well as recent advancements in methodology available to address unanswered research questions in this area.

INTRODUCTION

This review attempts to synthesize literature relevant to the impact of the common circumstance of transient anoxia on herbicide behavior in the soil environment, usually the result of temporary flooding. A variety of issues, such as herbicide function, carry-over damage to subsequent crops, or leaching to groundwater have necessitated a great deal of research on pesticide fate in the environment. Environmental fate of an herbicide can be expressed as the net effect of the compound's affinities for environmental compartments (Calamari and Barg, 1993), including the solid phase (in soil, this is generally controlled by sorption to either minerals or organic matter), the liquid phase (water solubility), the gas phase (volatility), and biota. Such partitioning is described by soil sorption coefficients (K_{OC} or K_D); water solubility; Henry's Constant (H); or the octanol/water partition coefficient (K_{OW}). These parameters say a great deal about the likely behavior of herbicides in the environment and are often used in predictive models.

Cells also take up xenobiotics from solution, which may lead to detoxification or biodegradation should the organism be so equipped, however, it is also important that even incompetent cells may take up xenobiotics, and in some cases, dead cells may have greater affinity for the substrates than live ones (Johnson and Kennedy, 1973; Voerman and Tammes, 1969). Permeability (or impermeability) of bacterial cells to ionic herbicides has been shown to influence herbicide uptake (Hultgren et al., 2000) as well as toxicity (Potera, 2003), and may also affect degradation kinetics at low concentrations or slow degradation rates.

Many environmental fate processes, including sorption, hydrolysis, volatilization, transport, irreversible sorption or binding of residues to the solid phase, and of course, degradation; may be directly or indirectly coupled (Sims and Cupples, 1999). Each of the fate processes may respond differently to environmental conditions, thus making the net effect on overall fate challenging to predict. The use of an integrated approach, in which several key fate processes are measured simultaneously, has proved helpful in determining which factors influence degradation rates over a range of environmental or soil conditions. Since microorganisms take up substrates from solution rather than from the sorbed phase (Sims and Cupples, 1999), desorption rate can control degradation rates for many compounds. Degradation studies employing several soils with a range of sorption properties often reveal strong correlations between empirical sorption and degradation measurements (Mervosh et al., 1995a, 1995b; O'Loughlin et al., 2000; Sims et al., 2009). The solution phase is usually depleted before the sorbed phase, resulting in an increase in apparent K_d over the course of the experiment (Mervosh et al., 1995a, 1995b), illustrating the importance of desorption hysteresis and diffusion constraints in unsaturated soil. Volatilization also competes with degradation for substrates in solution, thus conditions that impede degradation indirectly enhance volatilization as well.

THE SOIL PHYSICAL ENVIRONMENT

Soil can be simply generalized as containing solid space and pore space, the latter composed of liquid and gas phases, with the relative volumes of solid and pore space fixed (except for changes in bulk density caused by compaction or tillage), while the ratio of liquid and gas phase volumes within the pore space are highly variable. A greater proportion of gas phase volume favors transport of gases (including volatile pesticides) by diffusion, as the Fick's Law diffusion coefficient for gases, such as O_2 is generally about 10,000-fold greater through a volume of air than a volume of water. Conversely, non-volatile solutes do not move through the gas phase, thus undergo much slower diffusive transport as the proportion of liquid-filled pore space decreases. Thus, it is expected that resources that move primarily through the gas phase, such as O_2, are more available in dry soils, whereas non-volatile solutes are more available in wet soils. As a result, dry soils generally have an abundant oxygen supply due not only to rapid transport, but also reduced O_2 demand, as solutes become limiting for microbial activities. It follows that wet soils have limited O_2 supply owing to reduced transport of and increased demand for O_2 as a more abundant supply of solutes drives increased microbial activity. Unsaturated soils may contain anaerobic micro-sites, even if the soils appear well-drained. Sexstone et al. (1985) demonstrated the existence of anaerobic sites in soil aggregate centers using a Clark microelectrode. Aggregates as small as 6mm in diameter were occasionally found to contain anoxic centers, whereas those 4mm and less in diameter were oxic. Aggregates greater than10mm in diameter often had anaerobic centers. The occurrence of anaerobic centers was consistent with observed rates of respiration and oxygen diffusion. Nitrous oxide emissions appeared to be associated with anaerobic centers, which likely explains the occurrence of N_2O emissions from well-drained soils. Many agricultural soils have small aggregate sizes (2-4 mm) at the surface, owing in part to the effects of cultivation, thus larger, partially anoxic aggregates are more likely to occur below the surface. Similarly, apparently active aerobic organisms have been isolated from anoxic environments, such as a 2-picoline-degrading *Arthrobacter* sp. isolated from an iron-reducing aquifer contaminated with 2-picoline (O'Loughlin et al., 1999).

Transient water-logging conditions can occur in upland soils situated in positions subject to occasional saturation, as well as ephemeral wetlands, and may exist in a variety of situations, including arid or semi-arid environments. Thus, many soils bear evidence of transient anoxia (redox features), such as mottling (patchy color matrix, particularly yellow, brown and gray areas), segregation of iron or manganese minerals into nodules, or rust-colored (ferruginous) root channels or pore linings (Bryant et al., 2008) in a grey or yellowish matrix. Manganese and iron nodules (nodules generally contain oxides of both elements) have received considerable attention in the literature (Childs and Leslie, 1977; Liu et al., 2002) and have been characterized with respect to spatial organization of the oxides within the nodules (Dawson et al., 1985) and their functional significance, such as the potential to scavenge trace elements, including some substances of toxicological concern, such as Pb or Cr (Liu et al., 2002). In soils with ongoing alternation of saturation and drainage, nodules may either trap or release trace elements, depending on *in situ* pH and redox conditions (Cornua, et al., 2009). Efforts to characterize the degree of reducing conditions (indicators of reduction in soils, or IRIS) have involved a variety of approaches, most recently the use of synthetic iron oxides introduced as films on devices installed *in situ*, such as coated plastic tubes (Jenkinson and

Franzmeier, 2006; Rabenhorst and Burch, 2006). These efforts assist in delineating soils according to water regime, and may prove instructive in understanding the behavior of agricultural chemicals that undergo divergent fate scenarios under aerobic versus anoxic conditions, as frequently anoxic soils may be poised for rapid transition to anaerobic activities (Pett-Ridge and Firestone, 2005).

SOIL REDOX, TEMPORAL AND SPATIAL GRADIENTS

When O_2 is present, the equilibrium of chemical reactions involving oxygen is shifted toward oxidation, depleting reduced species. The electrochemical reactions involved are often described using the Nernst equation, which may be represented in abbreviated form as,

$$E = (E^o - 59\ mV/z)\ log10\ a_{Red}/a_{Ox} \qquad \text{Equation 1}$$

where E is the cell potential, or electromotive force, E^o standard cell potential under conditions of interest a_{Red} is the chemical activity for the reductant and a_{Ox} is the chemical activity oxidant, and z represents the moles of electrons transferred in the cell reaction. The overall state of the various redox reactions occurring simultaneously in soils can be observed by the use of a Pt electrode inserted into the soil matrix and connected to a volt meter (typically a pH meter measuring in millivolts). Electrical flow is accomplished by the inclusion of a reference electrode (often via a salt bridge consisting of saturated KCl in semisolid agar). The most common reference electrodes are Ag/AgCl (Ag^o and AgCl) and calomel (Hg^o and HgCl). The half cell reactions for these electrodes are as follows:

$$Ag^o\ Ag+ + e- \qquad \text{Equation 2}$$

$$Hg^o\ Hg^+ + e^- \qquad \text{Equation 3}$$

Redox data are generally normalized to a common reference (typically the standard hydrogen electrode, or SHE, which is impractical for field use). The correction factors for redox measurements taken with Ag/AgCl and calomel electrodes are +200 and + 250 mV respectively. When used in soil, Pt electrodes generally provide responses in the range of +600 mV to -400mV depending on electrode design and redox conditions, and are subject to a variety of interferences and periodic failures due to electrode construction, instrument design, and reactions with the environmental matrix (Rabenhorst and Burch, 2006). Measurements are reported relative to the SHE, which is defined as 0.0 mV.

Since many redox reactions involving soil minerals are also pH dependent, it is convenient to develop mineral stability diagrams that account for both pH and redox regime. For this purpose the electron activity, expressed as the negative log (pE) may be used in a modified Nernst equation (Eq 4), and this can be included in equilibrium expressions for mineral transformations that facilitate plotting concentrations of species as a function of pE and pH (Yong and Mulligan, 2004).

$$E = 59\ mV\ pE \qquad \text{Equation 4}$$

When soil becomes saturated, increased biological and chemical oxygen demand will result in the rapid depletion of O_2, which is only soluble at about 8 mg/Kg, and, as described above, is replenished at a much slower rate through water-filled pores. When oxygen demand exceeds supply, reduced species begin to accumulate, and an inserted Pt electrode will yield a more negative response. The electrode response generally continues to become more negative over time (until the driving force of oxygen demand, carbon, is depleted) and tends to be temporarily poised at particular redox ranges in a sequential pattern, due to the presence of specific electron acceptors that fuel heterotrophic activities. A variety of physiological controls and changes in physicochemical conditions drive succession in the microbial community, as different ecotypes compete for resources in the changing environment. During transient saturation, the pattern of dominant populations generally shifts from aerobic respiring organisms (poising E*h* at around 330mV) to those that can utilize as exogenous electron acceptors; NO_3^- (poising E*h* at around 220 mV), Mn(IV) poising E*h* at around 200mV, and finally Fe(III), poising E*h* at around 120 mV (correlation to observed Pt electrode reading may by poor in practice). Since iron is extremely plentiful in most soils, iron reduction continues over an extended period of time, during which fermentation (oxidation of organic compounds using an endogenous electron acceptor) becomes a competitive lifestyle. Eventually, as other electron acceptors are depleted and H_2 accumulates, sulfate-reducing bacteria (SRB) and archaea utilize SO_4^{2-} at around -150 mV and eventually methanogenic archaea begin to convert CO_2 or acetate to methane at around -250 mV in the last stage of the succession. The latter two stages generally dominate a flooded surface soil system only after extended submergence (weeks to months). Though some microsites may support sulfate reduction and methanogenesis under unsaturated or recently flooded conditions, transiently flooded soils are dominated by nitrate-reducing and iron-reducing conditions (Tor et al, 2000). The following equations summarize the dominant ecotypes, arranged in sequence of their peak activities after onset of saturation.

Aerobic respiration: ½ O2 + 2e- + 2H+ H2O Equation 5

Denitrification: $2NO_3^- + 12\ H^+ + 10e^-\ N_2 + 6H_2O$ Equation 6

Mn (IV) reduction: $MnO_2 + 4H^+ + 2e^-\ Mn^{2+} + 2H_2O$ Equation 7

Iron reduction: $Fe(OH)_3 + 3\ H^+ + 2e^-\ Fe^{2+} + 2H_2O$ Equation 8

Sulfate reduction: $SO_4^{2-} + 10H^+ + 8e^-\ H_2S + 4H_2O$ Equation 9

Methanogenesis: $CO_2 + 8\ H^+ + 8e^-\ CH_4 + 2\ H_2O$ Equation 10

This microbial succession is fairly predictable, and has been observed in a number of studies, particularly in rice agroecosystems, which received a great deal of attention in the 1960s (Patrick and Mahaptra, 1968) owing to the need to retain expensive added nitrogen fertilizers. Figure 1 depicts the expected temporal sequence of changes in concentration of electron acceptors or reduced products after a soil is flooded.

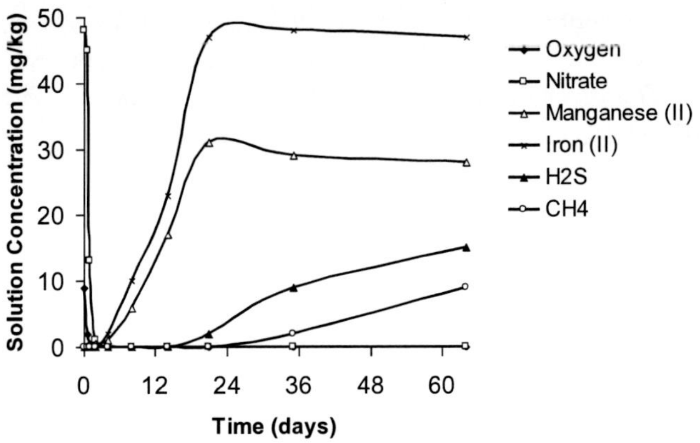

Figure 1. Temporal pattern for sequential reduction of electron acceptors assuming soil is inundated with water on day zero (adapted from Kannisery and Sims, 2011).

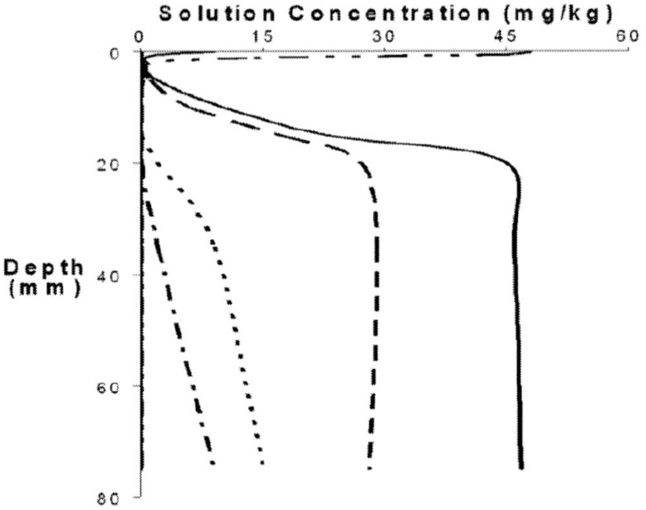

Figure 2. Spatial pattern for sequential reduction of electron acceptors assuming soil has been inundated with water long enough for methanogenesis to occur, that the water layer is shallow enough to deliver oxygen to the surface, and the oxygen demand is great enough to dissipate oxygen near the surface.

Sequential reduction follows not only a temporal pattern, but can be spatially stratified along O_2 supply/consumption gradients as well. Flooded rice agroecosystems have a relatively shallow water column, through which some O_2 penetrates, resulting in aerobic conditions at the surface, and reducing conditions stratified in space in the same order as the temporal changes in rodox that occur in the bulk soil after flooding. Patrick and Delaune (1972) demonstrated this by comparing redox potential measured with a Pt electrode to concentrations of electron acceptors or their microbial products as a function of depth in the surface of submerged soil. Moving downward through the soil, Mn(II) was the first reduced species encountered, followed by Fe(II) and then sulfide. The thickness of the oxidized layer increased with duration of flooding, likely owing to a decrease in O_2 demand as substrates were degraded. Thus, if the same succession described in Figure 1 is expressed on a spatial scale (with depth) in a rice field, a similar graph will describe the observed relationships (Figure 2).

In saturated soils, availability of electron acceptors for respiration and molecular oxygen for oxygenase-catalyzed reactions are likely the greatest constraints on net biodegradation kinetics. The pathways of degradation may change, owing to these constraints and energetics may be less favorable for oxidative metabolism without O_2 as a driver. However, bioavailability of soluble substrates is likely to improve when soils are saturated, though this effect likely increases competition among species that utilize common substrates. Saturation also facilitates cooperative relationships among microorganisms, which is a common feature of anaerobic communities, particularly under sulfate-reducing or methanogenic conditions (Gest, 2003). Carbon cycling under anoxia is generally perceived as being slower, exemplified by the tendency of natural materials, such as wood, to be preserved for extended periods of time in anaerobic environments. However, not all anaerobic processes operate slowly and some substrates are transformed more rapidly under anoxia (Loeffler et al., 2003). Moreover, for many years, anaerobic biodegradation received limited attention, owing, in part, to the greater challenge of conducting complex investigations in the containment needed to maintain rigorous anoxic conditions (given that human investigators require O_2). Since soils often contain microhabitats of differing redox conditions, it may be possible to see both strictly aerobic and strictly anaerobic degradation products occur in the same soil. In summary, in the absence of oxygen, organisms must be present that are equipped with appropriate metabolic machinery to transform xenobiotics without the aid of oxygenases and the overall community must be able to anaerobically process the resulting degradation products.

EXOGENOUS ELECTRON ACCEPTORS

Exogenous electron acceptors greatly improve the energetics of microbial metabolism over fermentative processes, thus the availability of electron acceptors in flooded soils is an important determinant of carbon cycling. Anaerobic biodegradation of herbicides thus may be stimulated by supplementing with specific electron acceptors, a hypothesis that is supported by a large body of literature with other substrates. For example, toluene has been shown to be susceptible to biodegradation coupled to nitrate (Zeyer et al., 1986; Major et al., 1988; Frazer et al, 1993), iron (Lovley et al, 1989) or sulfate (Haag et al., 1991, Beller et al., 1992), and similar reports are available for degradation of xylenes (Kuhn et al., 1985; Edwards et al., 1992) and benzoate (Taylor et al., 1970; Lovley and Phillips, 1988; Widdel, 1980) coupled with each of these electron acceptors. Conversely, the chloroacetamide herbicide, dimethenamid, exhibited similar fate regardless of the addition of electron acceptors or glucose (Crawford et al., 2002). All of these electron acceptors are expected to be available in most submerged soils, though their utilization generally will occur sequentially as described above.

Nitrate-reducing conditions. For herbicide metabolism, the most common role of O_2 at the substrate level is in halogen removal or ring activation/fission by either mono- or di-oxygenase attack. These functions may also be accomplished hydrolytically, and this is generally recognized experimentally when hydroxylated degradation products bear oxygen derived from water rather than air (using ^{18}O-labeled water). Nitrate is an excellent electron acceptor with a large change in free energy upon reduction, and numerous organisms are capable of taking advantage of this fact. However, nitrate is generally available in relatively limited quantities, even in fertilized soils, and can be depleted within one or two days of submergence of a surface soil (Tor et al., 2000), thus the overall impact of nitrate on herbicide fate may be transient. Nitrate inhibits the process of iron reduction, thus the initiation of iron-reducing conditions may be delayed when a greater supply of nitrate is available. Also, though the ability to use nitrate as an alternate electron acceptor to oxygen is widely distributed among the Eubacteria, coupling nitrate reduction to xenobiotic degradation requires a biodegradation mechanism that does not require molecular oxygen. Many denitrifiers function overall as aerobes that happen to be able to utilize nitrate as an alternative to O_2, and may not have been subjected to selection pressure to degrade a particular xenobiotic under anoxia. In an experiment that fits this general paradigm, Suflita et al. (1991) showed that the herbicide linuron was more rapidly degraded under either methanogenic or sulfate-reducing than nitrate reducing conditions in aquifer materials. Degradation of the herbicide mecoprop occurred at only low rates under either denitrifying or methanogenic sediments, whereas there was little or no evidence for degradation of atrazine, isoproturon, or metsulphuron-methyl in anoxic media (Larsen and J. Aamand, 2001). Gu et al. (1992) reported that atrazine was stable under nitrate-reducing conditions, however, nitrate reduction was also very slow in these microcosms (with the exception of one wetland soil), in contrast with results reported for Midwestern soils (Tor et al., 2000) or rice-producing soils that are commonly exposed to transient anoxia. Conversely, several bacteria have been shown unequivocally to degrade herbicides under denitrifying conditions. For example, *Ralstonia* sp. strain M91-3 (Crawford et al., 1998) and *Pseudomonas* sp strain ADP (Shapir, et al., 1998) can degrade atrazine using nitrate as an electron acceptor, though both organisms degrade atrazine far more rapidly in the presence of O_2. Crawford et al (1998) remains among the few studies to confirm the manner of nitrate disappearance (as N_2) in biodegradation coupled to denitrification by using $^{15}N_2$ headspace analysis. Degradation of bromoxynil (Preuβta, et al., 1995) was much more rapid under nitrate-reducing conditions (complete degradation in 32 days) than under aerobic conditions (no degradation within 32 days). The addition of acetate delayed onset of bromoxynil degradation under nitrate-reducing conditions (Preuβta, et al., 1995).

Wilber and Parkin (1995) found that transformation of both atrazine and alachlor in bioreactors was dependent upon supplying acetate as a co-metabolite. Incubations performed under aerobic, nitrate-reducing, sulfate-reducing, and methanogenic conditions resulted in biotransformation of both pesticides.

Negative results from studies performed *in situ* may sometimes be explained by the lack of competent indigenous organisms. Inoculation of anoxic sediments with *Pseudomonas* sp strain ADP enhanced atrazine degradation in nitrate-treated sediments (Shapir, et al., 1998), whereas inoculation of river sediments with *Ralstonia* sp. strain M91-3 had no effect on atrazine degradation, owing to elevated levels of indigenous degraders (Crawford et al., 1998).

Iron-reducing conditions. Typically, after complete depletion of nitrate, soils and sediments undergo iron-reducing conditions (Tor et al., 2000), which involves a significant change in community composition (Lueders and M. Friedrich, 2000; North et al., 2004). Several herbicides have been reported to undergo accelerated transformation in soils under iron-reducing conditions, though in most of these cases, it has not been clear that iron-reducing bacteria were directly involved in herbicide degradation. Even the use of sterile controls has been problematic, as autoclaving and gamma irradiation, the two most common means of producing sterile controls, liberate large concentrations of iron into solution, apparently disrupting iron minerals (Crawford et al., 2002).

Degradation of the herbicide acetochlor was similar under iron-reducing and methanogenic conditions in an anaerobic surface soil (Loor-Vela, 2003). Using cultures of *Comamonas koreensis* CY01, Wu et al. (2010) demonstrated iron reduction coupled to degradation of the herbicide, 2,4-dichlorophenoxyacetic acid (2,4-D). Several dinitroaniline herbicides, including trifluralin, pendimethalin, nitralin,and isopropalin (Tor et al., 2000; Wang and Arnold, 2003) appear to be transformed instead by microbially reduced iron minerals. Structural iron in nontronite (Tor et al., 2000) or surface-bound Fe(II) species in goethite suspensions (Wang and Arnold, 2003) as well as other naturally occurring reductants are able to reduce the nitro moieties in this class of chemicals, rapidly inactivating the compounds as herbicides. This is thought to be the primary reason that this herbicide class loses herbicidal function in low-lying areas of fields subject to ponding (Tor et al., 2000).

Reduction of ferruginous clays (by either chemical or microbial methods) were shown to enhance sorption of either atrazine or alachlor, likely due to changes in the surface acidity of the clays (Xu et al., 2001). Reduction of the clays promoted hydrolysis-dechlorination of atrazine, and resulted in accumulation of at least 14 alachlor degradation products. Oxidized or reduced and re-oxidized clays were much less effective adsorbants and had limited effect on degradation of either herbicide. Such biologically mediated abiotic transformation may be a promising approach for deactivating these compounds, though it is apparent that a great deal of the original herbicide may remain in the soil as unavailable bound residues.

Sulfate-reducing conditions. Sulfate becomes an important electron acceptor at low redox potentials that develop after prolonged anoxia and sulfate reduction is observed only under strict anaerobiosis. The sulfate-reducers are comprised of at least 220 species representing some 60 genera of bacteria and archaea (Barton Fauque, 2009).

They derive energy via oxidation of H_2 or organic compounds coupled to the reduction of oxidized sulfur compounds (such as sulfate, sulfite, thiosulfate, or elemental sulfur), and some may use a variety of other substrates, such as fumarate, nitrite, nitrate, Fe(III) or dimethyl sulfoxide. Sulfate-reducing bacteria (SRB) commonly produce hydrogen sulfide in concentrations that can have profound effects on the ecosystem. Sulfate reduction is energetically more favorable under acidic conditions, and the minimum redox potential (Eh) expected to accompany sulfate reduction decreases from around -50 to -200 mV as pH increases from 5 to 7 (Rabenhorst et al., 2006). Though transient anoxia in soils typically does not persist long enough for a substantial shift to sulfate-reducing conditions, sulfate reduction nonetheless may be detected after relatively short periods of flooding.

The expression of strictly anaerobic processes, such as sulfate reduction or methanogenesis is expected to be roughly proportional to the extent to which a soil undergoes occasional anoxia, even though populations of dormant methanogens and SRB can be detected in even the least likely environments, such as desert soils (Peters and Conrad, 1995). The majority of reports of herbicide degradation under sufate-reducing conditions involve test systems that are adapted to strict anoxia or have been equilibrated under anoxic conditions for a substantial period prior to or during the degradation studies. In surface soil pre-incubated with glucose under anoxic conditions, degradation of the herbicide acetochlor was found to be enhanced by the introduction of sulfate, decreasing the half life from 15 to 10 days (Loor-Vela, 2003). Kuhlmann and Kaczmarzcyk (1995) reported that the three auxin herbicides,

2,4-dichlorophenoxyacetic acid, (2,4-D), 2,4,5-trichlorophenoxyacetic acid (2,4,5-T), and 2-methyl-4-chlorophenoxyacetic acid (MCPA) persisted under sulfate-reducing conditions, degrading only after a substantial lag, though they were degraded without a lag under aerobic conditions.

Methanogenic conditions. As described above, methanogenic conditions may not develop substantially over the course of short-term flooding of normally unsaturated soils. To provide perspective, we will examine the fate of herbicides in acclimated methanogenic samples, e.g., river sediments. Lin et al. (2005) examined the fate of the herbicides, atrazine, cyanazine, and dicamba in anaerobically sampled river sediments incubated under methanogenic conditions. Only dicamba exhibited appreciable disappearance in less than a month.

The authors reported differences in behavior of the three herbicides, (atrazine proved more resistant to degradation than the other two herbicides over the course of the 300 day-incubation), and substantial disappearance of all of the substrates occurred in sterile samples, and followed similar kinetic patterns to the non-sterile samples.

Serial transfers to fresh medium eventually diluted out the matrix effects of the sediment (sterile controls no longer transformed the substrate) and resulted in enrichment of cultures expressing rapid degradation of cyanazine and dicamba degradation. Ramanand et al. (1993) reported that the herbicide, picloram (3,5,6-trichloro-4-amino-2-pyridinecarboxylic acid) was dehalogenated more readily under methanogenic conditions than when sulfate or nitrate was available as a terminal electron acceptor, and that the addition of sulfate to the incubation inhibited the process (an effect which could be overcome by the introduction of molybdate). The authors proposed that sulfate is preferred over the herbicide as an electron acceptor.

Reductive dehalogenation (halorespiration). Halorespiration involves the use of a halogenated substrate as an electron acceptor. Halorespiration is usually observed under strictly anaerobic conditions, and is thus most commonly associated with sulfate-reducing or methanogenic ecosystems.

The Myxobacterium, *Anaeromyxobacter dehalogenans*, is a unique halorespiring organisms that is also a metal reducer and carries out an unusual respiratory reduction of nitrate and nitrite to ammonia (Chee-Sanford et al., 2006). The term "halorespiring" is generally not used to describe the physiological state of an ecosystem as are "iron-reducing, sulfate-reducing, or methanogenic" (some halorespiring organisms belong to these groups) but is generally used to describe an organism or process.

Halorespiration likely evolved from the availability of naturally occurring chlorinated substratcs in an anaerobic environment. Under aerobic conditions, metabolism of halogenated compounds often involves oxygenase attack or hydrolytic removal of the halogen moiety (replacement with a hydroxyl group), and the favorability of this process decreases as electronegativity of the halogen decreases in the order iodine, bromine, chlorine and fluorine (Yong and Mulligan, 2004).

As the number of halogen substituents increases, the oxidation state of the carbon ring or backbone increases and oxidative removal becomes less favorable, and such substrates often persist in aerobic environments. Conversely halorespiration aka reductive dehalogenation (replacement of a halogen with a hydrogen), becomes energetically favorable under anoxia and is more favorable as the number of halogens increases.

Reductive dehalogenation has been demonstrated on a number of compounds under anaerobic conditions, such as chlorinated benzoates (Suflita et al., 1983) and the herbicides, 2,4,5, tichlorophenoxyacetic acid (Thayer, 1991) and methoxychlor (Baarschers et al., 1982).

Other examples of herbicides that have been shown to be subject to reductive dechlorination include alachor, metolachlor and propachlor (Stamper and Tuovinen, 1998). Both the bromine and iodine atoms have also been shown to be removed from certain herbicides (e.g. bromoxynil and ioxynil) by known chlorine respiring bacteria, such as *Desulfitobacterium chlororespirans* (Cupples et al., 2005).

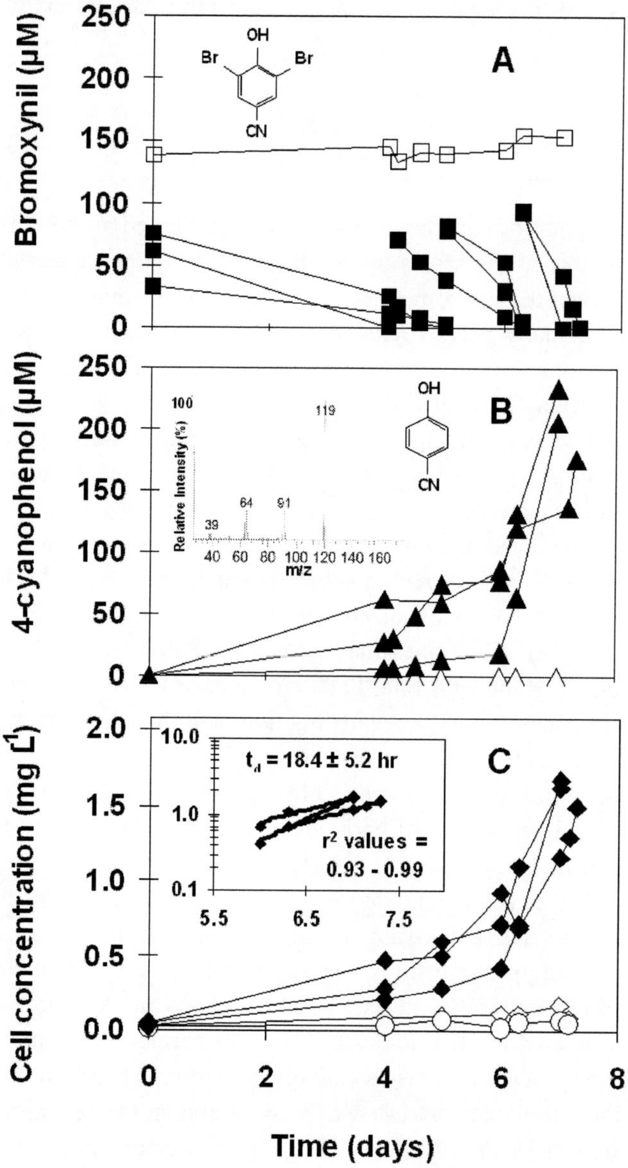

Figure 3. Bromoxynil (µM) removal in triplicate cultures (closed squares) and media control (open squares)(A), along with 4-cyanophenol (µM) formation in triplicate cultures (closed triangles) and media control (open triangles) (B). Increase in biomass concentration (mg L^{-1}) was determined by ^{14}C incorporation to new cells (closed diamonds) (C). No growth was observed when either cells (open circles) or bromoxynil were omitted (open diamonds). Insets are mass spectra of the metabolite (B) and doubling time (hr) during exponential growth (C). Copyright © American Society for Microbiology, Appl. Env. Micro. 71(7):3741-3746.

The process exhibited an initial lag phase but demonstrated immediate response after the system was dosed repeatedly (Figure 3). Sulfides accumulating in anaerobic systems have been found to react directly with some herbicides, opening the possibility of microbially-mediated abiotic transformations. Loch et al. (1999) and Stamper et al. (1997) described abiotic transformation mechanisms for degradation of the chloroacetanilide herbicides, alachlor, propachlor, and metolachlor by bisulfide, attributing the effect to dechlorination by HS- via an S_N2 reaction.

FUTURE DIRECTIONS

Process measurements for soils have largely been employed at the bulk scale, with much less information available at the scales upon which microbial processes likely vary (such as the aggregate scale), even though some types of process measurements on the aggregate scale have been possible for many years (Sexstone et al., 1985). Considerable advancement has been made in molecular biology tools for describing soil microbial populations and communities, or quantifying diversity, and some of these tools have been applied to herbicide degradation (Zablotowicz et al., 2006). However, until recently, directly linking phylogenetic descriptions to function *in situ* has been difficult. The advent of DNA and RNA-based stable isotope probing (SIP) has provided a powerful tool to identify organisms active in a particular process *in situ* without the need to cultivate the organisms involved (Sims, 2008). The general approach is to supply an ecosystem with a substrate (such as a herbicide) labeled with a very high level of isotopic enrichment of an element that will appear in the degrader's nucleic acids (generally ^{13}C or ^{15}N). The labled material is assimilated into the biomass of organisms active in the metabolism of the substrate. Labeled DNA or RNA are physically separated by differences in buoyant density (via ultracentrifugation) and the heavy fractions, containing the labeled nucleic acids, are subjected to molecular analysis. This method has been applied to a variety of hydrocarbons and simple substrates present in soil organic matter. Recently, several SIP studies have focused on the fate of herbicides, and have, for the first time, identified the active organisms *in situ*. Cupples et al. (2007) demonstrated the feasibility of using ^{15}N-labeled substrates for SIP in soils and determined the level of enrichment required to separate enriched bacteria of low native buoyant density (those with low G+C content) from un-enriched bacteria with high native buoyant density (those with high G+C content) using concentrations relevant to environment uses of herbicides. Cupples and Sims (2007) applied ^{13}C-DNA-SIP to the fate of the herbicide, 2,4-D in an agricultural soil. This study was the first to reveal the identity of the organisms actively degrading a herbicide *in situ*. Shaffer et al. (2010) tested the limitations of ^{15}N-DNA-SIP by applying the technique to the study of atrazine degradation in soils. Liu et al. (2011) demonstrated the dominance of Alphaproteobacteria among degraders of the herbicide, 2 - methyl - 4 - chlorophenoxyacetic acid (MCPA) in soils. Better tools (such as pyrosequencing) are now routinely available for identification of the active organisms, and this coupled with greater adoption of SIP techniques is rapidly increasing the level of knowledge of biodegradation *in situ*. Stable isotope probing has been applied to anaerobic systems (Kasai et al., 2006; Kunapuli et al., 2007) and is poised to give much greater insight into microbial succession and roles of different ecotypes during transient anoxia in soils.

SUMMARY

The bulk of the literature on herbicide fate under anoxia has been published within the last 15 years. Based on the current literature, it is apparent that transient surface soil saturation likely cycles surface soils predominantly through aerobic, nitrate-reducing, and iron-reducing conditions, while sulfate-reducing conditions and methanogenesis are more likely to become dominant process only in longer-term flooding events. Though data are limited, it is clear that some herbicides may be transformed quite rapidly under transient reducing conditions, and in the case of microbially-induced abiotic transformations (such as reaction of herbicides with reduced minerals), the parent compound may be dissipated much faster than under aerobic conditions. Projected changes in future rainfall patterns (such as for the American Midwest) may thus have profound influences on the function of soil-applied herbicides. The advent of new tools in molecular biology, and especially DNA- and RNA-based stable isotope probing are rapidly increasing our understanding of herbicide microbiology and are presently the tools of choice in following the complex succession of active organisms expected to occur in the cycling of soils through different water regimes.

REFERENCES

Baarschers, W.H., Bharath, AI, Elvish, J, and Davies, M. (1982). The biodegradation of methoxychlor by *Klebsiella pneumonia*. *Can. J. Microbiol. 28*:176-179.

Barton, L.L. and Fauque, G.D. (2009). Biochemistry, physiology and biotechnology of sulfate-reducing bacteria. *Advances in Applied Microbiology 58*: 41-98.

Beller, H., Grbić-Galić, D., and Reinhard, M. (1992). Microbial degradation of toluene under sulfate-reducing conditions and the influence of iron on the process. *Appl. Environ. Microbiol. 58*:786-793.

Bryant, K.L., Wilson, P.R., Biggs, A.J.W., Brough, D.M., and Burgess, J.W. (2008). Soil indicators of Queensland wetlands: Statewide assessment and methodology. *Department of Natural Resources and Water, Brisbane*.

Calamari, D. and Barg, U. (1993). Hazard assessment of agricultural chemicals by simple simulation models. In: *Prevention of water pollution by agriculture and related activities*. Proceedings of the FAO Expert Consultation, Santiago, Chile, 20-23 Oct. 1992. Water Report 1. FAO, Rome. pp. 207-222.

Chee-Sanford, J.C., Sanford, R.A., Loffler, F.E., Thomas, S.H., Sims, G.K. (2006). Investigating anaerobic microbial processes in agricultural soils using Anaeromyxobacter dehalogenans as a cosmopolitan model. *Abstracts of the International Soc. for Microbial Ecology*. 11:152.

Childs, C.W. and Leslie, D.M. (1977). Inter-element relationships in iron-manganese concretions from a catenary sequence of yellow-grey earth soils in loess. *Soil Science, 123*(6): 369-376.

Cornua, S., Cattlea, J.A., Samouëliana, A., Laveufa, C., Guilhermea, L.R.G., Albérice, P. (2009). Impact of redox cycles on Mn, Fe, Co and Pb in nodules. *Soil Science Society of America Journal. 73*(4):1231-1241.

Crawford, J.J., Sims, G.K., Mulvaney, R.L., and Radosevich, M. (1998). Biodegradation of atrazine under denitrifying conditions. *Appl. Microbiol. Biotechnol. 49*:618-623.

Crawford, J.J., Sims, G.K., Simmons, F.W., Wax, L.M., and Freedman, D.L. (2002). Dissipation of the herbicide (14C) dimethenamid under anaerobic aquatic conditions in flooded soil microcosms. J. *Agric. Food. Chem. 50*(6): 1483-1491.

Cupples, A.M. and Sims, G.K. (2007). Identification of in situ 2,4-dichlorophenoxyacetic acid-degrading soil microorganisms using DNA-stable isotope probing. *Soil Biology and Biochemistry 39*: 232-238.

Cupples, A.M., Sanford, R.A. and Sims, G.K. (2005). Dehalogenation of bromoxynil (3,5-bibromo-4-hydroxybenzonitrile) and ioxynil (3,5-di-iodino-4-hydroxybenzonitrile) by *Desulfitobacterium chlororespirans*. *Appl. Env. Micro. 71*(7):3741-3746.

Cupples, A.M., Shaffer, E.A. Chee-Sanford, J.C. and Sims, G.K. (2007). DNA buoyant density shifts during ^{15}N DNA stable isotope probing. *Microbiological Res. 162*:328-334.

Dawson, B.S.W., Fergusson, J.E., Campbell, A.S., and Cutler, E.J.B. (1985). Distribution of elements in some Fe-Mn nodules and an iron-pan in some gley soils of New Zealand. *Geoderma. 35*:127-143.

Edwards, E.A., Wills, L.E., Reinhard, M., and Grbić-Galić, D. (1992). Anaerobic degradation of toluene and xylene by aquifer microorganisms under sulfate-reducing conditions. *Appl. Environ. Microbiol. 58*:794-800.

Frazer, A.C., Ling, W., and Young, L.Y. (1993). Substrate induction and metabolic accumulation during anaerobic toluene utilization by the denitrifying stain T1. *Appl. Environ. Microbiol. 59*:3157-3160.

Gest, H. (2003). Anaerobes in the recycling of elements in the biosphere. Ljungdahl, L. (Ed.) *Biochemistry and physiology of anaerobic bacteria*. (pp. 4-10). Springer-Verlag, New York.

Gomez, A.M., Yannarell, A.C., Sims, G.K., Cadavid-Resterpoa, G., and Herrera, C.X.M. (2011). Characterization of bacterial diversity at different depths in the Moravia Hill Landfill site at Medellín, Colombia. *Soil Biology and Biochemistry 43*:1275-1284.

Gu, J.-D., Berry, D.F., Taraban, R.H, Martens, D.C., Walker, Jr., H.L., and Edmonds, W.J. (1992). Biodegradability of Atrazine, Cyanazine, and Dicamba in Wetland Soils. *Virginia Water Resources Research Center Bulletin 172*. Virginia Polytechnic Institute and State University, Blacksburg.

Haag, F., Reinhard, M., and McCarty, P.L. (1991). Degradation of toluene and *p*-xylene in anaerobic microcosms: Evidence for sulfate as a terminal electron acceptor. *Environ. Tox Chem. 10*: 1379-1389.

Hultgren, R.P., Hudson, R.J. and Sims, G.K. (2002). Effects of soil pH and soil water content on prosulfuron dissipation. *J. Agric. Food Chem. 5* (11): 3236-3243.

Jenkinson, B.J. and Franzmeier D.P. (2006). Development and evaluation of Fe-coated tubes that indicate reduction in soils. *Soil Science Society America Journal. 70*:183–191.

Johnson, B.T., and Kennedy, J.O. (1973). Biomagnification of p.p. DDT and methoxychlor by bacteria. *Appl. Environ. Microbiol. 26*:66-71.

Kanissery, R.G., and Sims, G.K. (2011). Biostimulation for the enhanced degradation of herbicides in soil. *Applied and Environmental Soil Science. 2011*, Article ID 843450, doi:10.1155/2011/843450.

Kasai, Y., Takahata, Y., Manefield, M., and Watanabe, K. (2006). RNA-based stable isotope probing and isolation of anaerobic benzene-degrading bacteria from gasoline-contaminated groundwater. *Appl. Environ. Microbiol. 72*(5): 3586-3592.

Kuhlmann, B., and Kaczmarzcyk, B. (1995). Biodegradation of the herbicides 2,4-dichlorophenoxyacetic acid, 2,4,5-trichlorophenoxyacetic acid, and 2-methyl-4-chlorophenoxyacetic acid in a sulfate-reducing aquifer. *Environmental Toxicology and Water Quality. 10*(2):119–125.

Kuhn, E.P., Colberg, P.J., Schnoor, J.L., Wanner, O., Zehnder, A.J.B., and Schwartzenbach, R.P. (1985). Microbial transformation of substituted benzenes during infiltration of river water to ground water: Laboratory column studies. *Environ. Sci. Technol. 19*:961-968.

Kunapuli, U., Lueders, T., and Meckenstock, R.U. (2007). The use of stable isotope probing to identify key iron-reducing microorganisms involved in anaerobic benzene degradation. *The ISME Journal. 1*:643–653.

Larsen, L. and Aamand, J. (2001) Degradation of herbicides in two sandy aquifers under different redox conditions. *Chemosphere. 44*(2):231–236).

Lin, C., Gu, J.-G., Qiao, C., Duan, S. and. Gu, J.D. (2006). Degradability of atrazine, cyanazine, and dicamba in methanogenic enrichment culture microcosms using sediment from the Pearl River of Southern China. *Biol Fertil Soils. 42*:395–401.

Liu, F., Colombo, C., Adamo, P., He, J.Z. and Violante, A. (2002). Trace elements in manganese-iron nodules from a Chinese Alfisol. *Soil Science Soc. Am. J.. 66*:661-670.

Liu, Y.J., Liu, S.J., Drake, H.L., and Horn, M.A. (2011). Alphaproteobacteria dominate active 2‑methyl‑4‑chlorophenoxyacetic acid herbicide degraders in agriculturalmethyl‑4‑chlorophenoxyacetic acid herbicide degraders in agricultural soil and drilosphere. Environ. Microbiol. 13(4):991-1009.

Loch, A.R., Traina, S.J., and Chin, Y.-P..(1999). Abiotic degradation of chloroacetanilide herbicides by bisulfide. *Extended Abstracts of the American Chemical Society. 39*(1): 51-53.

Loeffler, F.E., Cole, J.R., Ritalahti, K.M., and Tiedje, J.M. (2003). Diversity of dechlorinating bacteria. In Haggblom, M.M., and Bossert, I.D. (Eds.). *Dehaologenation: Microbial processes and environmental applications*. Kluwer Academic Publishers, Dordrecht, The Netherlands.

Loor-Vela, S.X., Crawford-Simmons, J.J., Simmons, F.W., and Raskin, L. (2003). Dissipation of [(14)C]acetochlor herbicide under anaerobic aquatic conditions in flooded soil microcosms. *J. Agric. Food Chem. 51*(23):6767-6773.

Lovley, D.R., and Phillips, E.P.J. (1988). Novel mode of microbial energy metabolism: Organic carbon oxidation coupled to dissimilatory reduction of iron or manganese. *Appl. Environ. Microbiol. 54*:1472-1480.

Lovley, D.R., Baedeker, M.J., Lonergan, D.J., Cozzarelli, I.M., Phillips, E.P.J., and Siegel, D.I. (1989). Oxidation of aromatic contaminants coupled to microbial iron reduction. *Nature. 329*:297-299.

Lueders, T. and Friedrich, M. (2000). Archaeal population dynamics during sequential reduction processes in rice field soil. *Applied and Environmental Microbiology. 66*: 2732–2742.

Major, D.W., Mayfield, C.I., and Barker, J.F. (1988). Biotransformation of benzene by denitrification in aquifer sand. *Ground Water. 26*:8-14.

Mervosh, T.L., Sims, G.K., and Stoller, E.W. (1995). Clomazone fate in soil as affected by microbial activity, temperature, and soil moisture. *J. Agric. Food Chem. 43*:537-543.

Mervosh, T.L., Sims, G.K., Stoller, E.W., and Ellsworth, T.R. (1995). Clomazone sorption in soil: Incubation time, temperature, and soil moisture effects. *J. Agric. Food Chem. 43*:2295-2300.

North, N.N., Dollhopf, S.L., Petrie, L., Istok, J.D., Balkwill, D.L., and Kostka, J.E. (2004). Change in bacterial community structure during in situ biostimulation of subsurface sediment co-contaminated with uranium and nitrate. *Applied and Environmental Microbiology. 70*(8):4911–4920.

O'Loughlin, E. J., Sims, G.K. and Traina, S.J. (1999). Biodegradation of 2-methyl, 2-ethyl, and 2-hydroxypyridine by an *Arthrobacter sp.* isolated from subsurface sediment. *Biodegradation 10*:93-104.

O'Loughlin, E.J, Traina, S.J., and Sims, G.K. (2000). Effects of sorption on the biodegradation of 2-methylpyridine in aqueous suspensions of reference clay minerals. *Environ. Toxicol. and Chem. 19*:2168-2174.

Patrick, W.H. and Delaune, R.D. (1972). Characterization of the oxidized and reduced zones in flooded soil. *Soil Science Society of America Journal 36*(4): 573-576.

Patrick, W.H., and Mahaptra, I.C. (1968). Transformation and availability to rice of nitrogen and phosphorus in waterlogged soils. *Adv. Agron. 20*:323-359.

Peters, V. and Conrad, R. (1995) Methanogenic and other strictly anaerobic bacteria in desert soil and other oxic soils. *Appl. Environ. Microbiol. 61*:1673-1676.

Pett-Ridge, J. and Firestone, M.K. (2005). Redox fluctuation structures: Microbial communities in a wet tropical soil. *Appl. Environ. Microbiol. 71*(11): 6998–7007.

Potera, R. M. (2003). Effects of acetolactate synthase inhibiting herbicides on soil microorganisms. *University of Illinois at Urbana-Champaign.*

Preuβta, G, Zullei-seiberta, N., Heimlichb,F., Nolte, J. (1995). Degradation of the herbicide bromoxynil in batch cultures under groundwater conditions. *International Journal of Environmental Analytical Chemistry. 58*: 207-213.

Rabenhorst M.C. and Burch, S.N. (2006). Synthetic iron oxides as an indicator of reduction in soils (IRIS). *Soil Science Society America Journal 70*: 1227–1236.

Rabenhorst, M.C., Fanning, D.S., and Burch, S.N. (2006). Acid sulfate soils: Formation. In. Lal, R. (Ed.). *Encyclopedia of soil science*. (pp. 20-24) CRC Press Taylor Francis Group Boca Raton, Florida, USA.

Rabenhorst, M.C., Hively, W.D., and James, B.R. (2009). Measurements of soil redox potential. *Soil Sci. Soc. Am. J. 73*(2) 668-674.

Ramanand, K., Nagarajan, A., and Suflita, J.M. (1993). Reductive dechlorination of the nitrogen heterocyclic herbicide picloram. *Appl. Environ. Microbiol. 59*(7): 2251–2256.

Sexstone, A.J., Revsbech, N.P., Parkin, T.B., and Tiedje, J.M. (1985). Direct measurement of oxygen profiles and denitrification rates in soil aggregates. *Soil Science Society of America Journal. 49*(3): 645-651.

Shaffer, E.A., Sims, G.K., Cupples, A.M, Smyth, C., Chee-Sanford, J., and. Skinner, A. (2010). Atrazine biodegradation in a Cisne soil exposed to a major spill. *International Journal of Soil, Sediment and Water. 3*(Issue 2, Article 5):1-26.

Shapir, N., Mandelbaum, R.T., and Jacobsen, G.S. (1998). Rapid atrazine mineralization under denitrifying conditions by *Pseudomonas* sp. strain ADP in aquifer sediments. *Environmental Science and Technology. 32*(23):3789–3792.

Sims, G.K. (2008). Stable isotope probing to investigate microbial function in soil. *Recent Research Developments in Soil Science. 2*(2007): 64-85.

Sims, G.K. and Cupples, A.M. (1999). Factors controlling degradation of pesticides in soil. *Pesticide Science 55*:598-601.

Sims, G.K., Taylor-Lovell, S. Tarr, G. and Maskel, S. (2009). Role of sorption and degradation in the herbicidal function of isoxaflutole. *Pest Management Science 65*(7):805-810.

Stamper, D.M. and Tuovinen, O.H. (1998). Biodegradation of the acetanilide herbicides alachlor, metolachlor, and propachlor. *Critical Reviews in Microbiology. 24(*1):1–22.

Stamper, D.M., Traina, S.J., and Tuovinen, O.H. (1997). Anaerobic transformation of alachlor, propachlor and metolachlor with sulfide. *J. Environ. Qual. 26*:488-494.

Suflita, J.M., Ramanand, K., and Adrien, N. (1991).Anaerobic biotransformation of halogenated pesticides in aquifer slurries. In Baker, R.A. (Ed.) *Organic substances in water, Volume 3: Biological.* (pp. 199-210). Lewis Publishers, Chelsea, Michigan.

Suflita, J.M., Robinson, J.A. and Tiedje, J.M. (1983). Kinetics of microbial dehologenation of haloaromatic substrates in methanogenic environments. *Appl. Environ. Microbiol. 45:*1466-1473.

Thayer, A.M. (1991). Bioremediation: Innovative technology for cleaning up hazardous waste. *Chem. Eng. News. 69*(34):23-44.

Tor, J., Xu, C. Stucki, J.M., Wander, M., and Sims G.K. (2000). Trifluralin degradation under micro-biologically induced nitrate and Fe(III) reducing conditions. *Env. Sci. Tech. 34*:3148-3152.

Voerman, S., and Tammes, R.M.C. (1969). Adsorption and desorption of lindane and dieldrin by yeast. *Bull. Environ. Contam. Toxicol. 4*:271-277.

Wang, S., and Arnold, W.A. (2003). Abiotic reduction of dinitroaniline herbicides. *Water Research. 37*(17):4191–4201.

Widdel, F. (1980). Anaerobic degradation of fatty acids and benzoic acid by newly isolated types of sulfate-reducing bacteria. Doctoral Dissertation, Georg-August-Universität, Göttengen.

Wilber, G.G., and Parkin, G.F. (1995). Kinetics of alachlor and atrazine biotransformation under various electron acceptor conditions. *Environ. Toxicol. Chem. 14*:237-244.

Wu, C.Y., Zhuang, L.S., Zhou, G., Li, F.B., and Li, X.M. (2010). Fe(III)-enhanced anaerobic transformation of 2,4-dichlorophenoxyacetic acid by an iron-reducing bacterium *Comamonas koreensis* CY01. *FEMS Microbiology Ecology. 71*(1):106–113.

Xu, J., Stucki, J.W., Wu, J., Kostka, J. and Sims, G.K. (2001). Fate of atrazine and alachlor in redox-treated ferruginous smectite. *Env. Tox. and Chem. 20*: 2717-2724.

Yong, R.N., and Mulligan, C.N. (2004). Natural attenuation of contaminants in soils. Lewis Publishers. Boca Raton, Florida, USA.

Zablotowicz, R.M., Weaver, M.A., and Locke, M.A. (2006). Microbial adaptation for accelerated atrazine mineralization/degradation in Mississippi Delta soils. *Weed Science 54*(3):538-547.

Zeyer, J., Kuhn, E.P., and Schwartzenbach, R.P. (1986). Rapid microbial mineralization of toluene and 1,3-dimethylbenzene in the absence of molecular oxygen. *Appl. Environ. Microbiol. 52*:944-947.

In: Xenobiotics: New Research
Editors: Saul F. Castaneda and Mauro L. Emerson
ISBN: 978-1-61942-616-0

Chapter 5

Correction of Mutagenic and Pro Oxidant Activity of Heavy Metals

A. R. Gutnikova, B. A. Saidkhanov, M. S. Gildieva, N. Kh. Ablyaeva, and I. V. Kosnikova
V. Vakhidov Republican Specialized Center of Surgery,
Institute of Genetics and Experimental Plant Biology of ASc. RU, Uzbekistan

Abstract

Heavy metals, anthropogenic toxicants, can penetrate into the human organism in tiny amounts through food and water and then accumulate, promoting oppression of mono-oxygenase systems of a liver and possesses pro-oxidative and mutagen activity In this paper, pathological disorders in liver due to heavy metals effects and their treatment have been investigated. The obtained data has confirmed the fact that in activation and deactivation of the mutagens the big role is played by free radicals, condition MOS and antioxidative organism systems. It was shown that the course of the entero-sorption therapy by a citric pectin sorbent in a combination with antioxidative phyto-preparation provides reducing of intensity of the generated pathological variations.

Introduction

The development of the living world occurs in permanent contact with the environment. According to Vernadsky biogeochemical theory there exists " biogenic migration of atoms" through the chain air →soil →water→ food→ man, and as a result practically all elements surrounding a man in environment penetrate the organism to a greater or smaller degree [7;8;20]. Consuming nutrition and water promote organism's filling with chemical elements. The element's concentration in living substance is directly proportional to its content in the surroundings with due regard for their combinations solubility. In other words the chemical composition of the organism is determined by the environment's composition. The increasing nature of the anthropogenic chemical influence all over the world is due to the existence of toxicants in the air space and in food-stuffs. The tendency of increasing content of heavy metal's combinations in the basic food products revealed by a member of investigators in of special importance.

The distinctive feature of heavy metals (H M) as ecopollutants is their stability in the environment, high toxic ability for living organisms and under relatively low concentrations and their bio-accumulative ability [10;15]. A lot of HM are inductors of oxidizing stress [1, 11;17], and the forming products of free-radical oxidation in their turn can initiate mutagenesis in cells [4,9;12;14]. Under conditions when the organism's exposition to HM is abnormal the urgent problem is searching of means not only reducing the toxic influence on the organism but also possessing antioxidant and anti mutagenic properties. As regards detoxification the most perspective entero-sorbents are to be, the ones obtained from different food fibers as well as various phytoherbs possessing the proved antioxidant properties. Quite a number of investigations are dedicated to the studies on efficiency and selection of such antitoxic bio preparations [3,6,13;18;20]. The anti mutagenic properties of such complexes as well as the interpretation of their advisable use for the pathological process arresting including the mutagenic effect of HM have been studied to a less degree. In accordance to our previous investigations it was determined that Hepamal preparation representing an oil phytoherb extract containing the flowers of immortelle and costmary and sweetbrier fruit had worked antioxidant properties [5]. It's using together with pectin entero-sorbent leads to regression of the pathological process during intoxication by HM [2].

The aim of the present investigation is to study the influence of heavy metal mixture on the lipoperoxidation process, the activity of the liver's mono oxigenase system and mutagenesis inside the cells of red marrow, and also to determine the efficiency of the proposed tactics for the pathological process of arresting.

EXPERIMENTAL

The investigations were conducted using 60 white mongrel rats with the initial mass equal to 180-190g., with the standard diet according to the established worm. The animals were divided into 3 groups: intact, HM intoxication was modeled by means of intraperitoneum injection of water suspension obtained from copper, manganese, molybdenum and chromium salts typical for the area influenced by Almalyk Mining Metallurgical Group of Enterprises, once in two days during 4 weeks. The matter content (mg/kg) was: $CuSO_4$-60, $KMnO_4$-11,2, $(NH_4)_2MoO_4$-10, $K_2Cr O_7$-1,19. The correction of the forming pathological disturbances was realized by means of entero-sorbtion and antioxidant therapy combination which was begun after the intoxication manifestation. The correction was conducted every day during 3 weeks. The citric pectin with the molecular mass of 70 thousand, the etherification degree of 50%, the carboxyl content of 0,6% was used as a sorbent, which was injected once a day through a probe in the dose of 0,5g per 100g of an animal's mass 1 hour before feeding. Hepamal, injected per os 2 hours after feeding once a day in the dose of 1ml/100gof the body mass, was used as an antioxidant. After the completion of the process modeling and the treatment termination the animals of all groups were killed by a momentary decapitation and then the process of blood sampling was carried out in order to evaluate the state of pro- and antioxidant system and liver tissue for the purpose of P450 and B5 cytochrome determination. Some of animals (in five animals from every group) which red marrow cells were extracted for analysis, 2-2,5 hours before killing were injected with 0,025% colchicines solution intraperitoneumly. The marrow cells were analyzed (in100 cells from every tested animal) with typical high level of their mitotic activity. The cells in metaphase were analyzed. The mutagenic activity was determined according to C.Ford & Y. Hamerton method (1994) [19] which is based on the registration of obvious chromosome disturbance in cells in metaphase on the registration of obvious chromosome disturbance in cells in metaphase stage. A solvent was used as a negative control. The analysis of cells with metaphase plates was carried out by using of Leica microscope with ocular 10x, objective 100x. Unbroken cells with good chromosome dispersion were selected for the analysis. Every metaphase plate was the presence of chromosome aberrations in it: fragments, deletions, exchanges, plural aberrations.

Table 1. Changes in metabolic activity of MOS and antioxidative system caused by heavy metal poisoning and after therapy course, n 45

Index	Group 1. Control (Healthy)	Group 2. – intoxication by heavy metal, P_{1-2}	Group3. – after therapy course P_{2-3} P_{1-3}
Index in liver tissue:			
Cytochrome P450, nmol mg^{-1} of protein	0,80 ± 0,01	0,51±0,03 <0,001	0,84±0,07 <0,02 >0,05
Cytochrome B5, nmol mg^{-1} of protein	0,63±0,01	0,40±0,03 <0,001	0,66±0,05 <0,02 >0,05
Catalase, a. u.	4,7±0,8	3,7±0,7 >0,05	7,5±0,9 <0,02 <0,05
Glutathione reductase, a. u.	195±13	163±7 <0,05	234±3,6 <0,001 <0,05
Index in blood serum:			
MDA, μmol L^{-1}	2,5±0,02	3,5±0,1 <0,001	2,22±0,1 <0,01 >0,05
AOA, %	31,4±0,8	15,7±0,9 <0,001	30,8±0,5 <0,001 >0,05
Catalase, a. u.	24,3±2,8	17,3±1,4 <0,05	21,7 ±3,1 >0,05 >0,05
Glutathione reductase, a. U.	13,6 ±1,9	7,4±2,0 <0,05	20,7±2,0 <0,02 <0,05

Results and Discussion

P-450-cytochrome-dependent mono oxygenize system (MOS) is known to be the main enzyme system maintaining the inner chemical homeostasis and responsible for the inactivation of alien low molecular compounds.

As appears from the figures presented in Table 1, the injection of HM results in the obvious inhibiting of MOS. P450 and B5 cytochrome content is decreased by more than 36%, this indicating the exhausting of reserved and breaching if the compensator detoxicative mechanisms of liver (Table 1). It is typical that these changes take place together with the considerable activation of the process of lipid-peroxide oxidation (POL) that was confirmed by the increasing MDA concentration by 40%, and it promotes the exhausting of antioxidant of antioxidant activity of the serum (AOA) is decreased twice, the activity of Catalase and Glutathione reductase (GR) is reduced by 28% and 46%, correspondingly. The analogous dynamics is observed in the liver tissue too. The activity of AOP enzymes is decreased: for Catalase- by 21%, for Glutathione reductase- by 16%.

The analysis of the given data (Table2) showed that after incorporation of the metal line mixture to animals the number of pathological mitosis is increased. In our experiments this phenomenon was observed in 60,4 % of the blast cells under investigation (from 20% up to 90% of cells). Those were mainly K-mitosis (colchicine's mitosis) (Figures 1,2). This mitosis pathology is connected with the damage of the mitotic apparatus and its peculiar feature is the blockage of cell-division during metaphase. K-mitosis were found in several morphological variants depending on the damage extent of the mitotic apparatus and chromosomes: gluing of chromosomes with a lump for motion, hyper helix formation, dispersion of chromosomes, asymmetrical mitosis. The outcome of K-mitosis is the cells destruction or formation of hypo- and polyploidy cells. The mitotic index of marrow cells in this group of animals was 3 times less than in control, and only in 10 %- 40% of cells normal metaphase plates were found. In this connection the level of chromosome aberration was not very high either, 6,0% on average (from 4% up to 12%), that in negative control (1%). Only one animal from this group had all the data, except the mitotic index, which were much less than the other animals, with the mitotic index at the negative control level (6,4%).Thus, the conducted scientific researchers showed that intoxication by the HM mixture under investigation results in marked tension of the biotransformative processes in liver. The observed POL inductions, the decreasing of AOP activity induce the activation of mutagens.

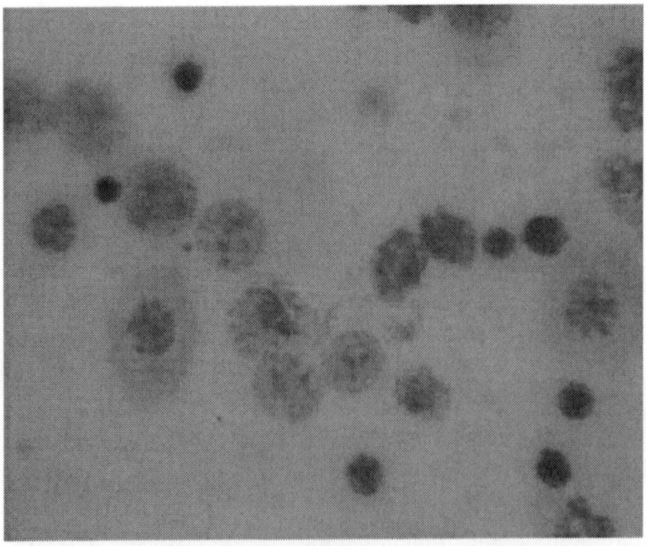

Figure 1. Cells of a red marrow of healthy rats: normal metaphase plates, absence of pathological mitoses, a high mitotic index.

Table 2. Cytogenetic investigation of red morrow cells of rats caused by heavy metal intoxication and after therapy course, n 15

Index	Group 1- control (healthy)	Group 2.- intoxication by heavy metal P_{1-2}	Group 3.- after therapy course P_{2-3} P_{1-3}
Mitotic index, %	9,6±0,9	3,96±0,7 <0,05	8,0±0,7 <0,05 >0,05
Number of metaphase	400	500	500
Number of aberrant metaphase	1	15	3
Number of chromosome aberrations	1±0,5	6,0±0,6 <0,05	1,2±0,4 <0,05 >0,05
Hypo- and polyploidy	1,0±0,05	19,7±3,8 <0,05	2,0±0,05 <0,05 >0,05
K-mitosis, %	0	50,7±3,5 <0,05	8,0±0,7 <0,05 <0,05
Mitosis pathology, %	0	73,3±1,2 <0,05	10,0±0,2 <0,05 <0,05

A number of measures aimed in reducing of HM cytotoxic effects were selected in order to arrest the formed pathological changes. These measures combine entero-sorbtion detoxification with antioxidant therapy. It was ascertained that after medical treatment the metabolite activity of MOS was restored within the limits of physiological standard, that was indicated by the increasing of P450 and B5 cytochrome concentration up to the level of intact values. It coincided with the arresting of POL process and increasing of the organism's antioxidant status. MDA concentration was reduced 1,6 times with the considerable growth of AOP enzyme activity. The increase of catalase activity in blood serum was equal to 24%, glutathione reductase activity and AOA was 2,7 times and 2 times higher, correspondingly. The investigate enzyme activity in the liver tissue was also increased: for catalase -twice, for glutathione reductase –by 1,4 times. It is characteristic that both values were higher than the level of the intact values thus indicating the stimulating influence of the conducted therapy towards AOP system.

All data concerning mutagenic activity and approached the healthy animals' data changed too. Thus the amount of pathological mitosis animals had was decreased to 2,5% (from 0 up to 8%). K-mitosis disappeared, hypo- and polyploidy cells as well as the amount of chromosome aberrations were at the intact values level (Figure 3). So the investigation of chromosome aberration in red morrow cells of rats ascertains that introduction of heavy metal salts induced mutagenesis. It is indicated by the increased amount of pathological mitosis, decreased amount of chromosome aberrations and mitotic index.

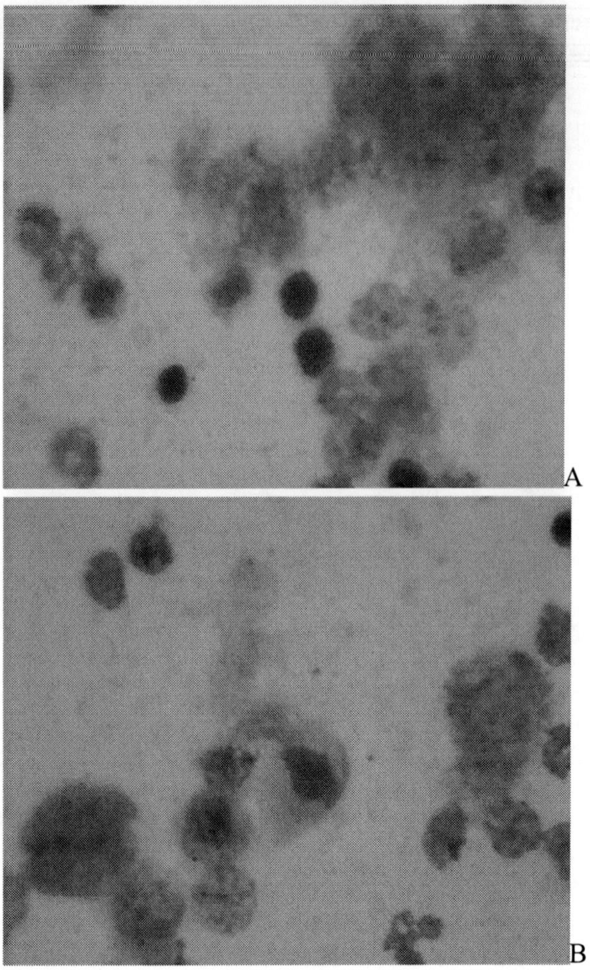

Figure 2. Cells of a red marrow of rats with intoxication's syndrome induced by salts of heavy metals. A – In the center - a cell with K-mitoses and a hollow metaphase; B- at the left and on the right - the cell with dispersion of chromosomes, in the center hyper spiralization of chromosomes in a metaphase.

The obtained data confirmed the fact that free radicals, organism's MOS and AOP system state were of great importance in activation and inactivation of mutagens. Incorporation of the HM mixture under investigation leads to disturbance of cells' reproduction and consequently results in their physiological and reparative regeneration. The damage of the mitotic apparatus and the blockage of cell-division during metaphase that was indicated by the increased amount of K-mitosis should be considered as the main peculiar feature. The obtained results are in coincidence with the other the original cause or the initial stage of the induced mutagenesis activation are the products of free – radical reactions provocation the damage of DNA- molecules in cells [4]. The course of combined antioxidant and enterosorbtion therapy secured arresting of the pathological process owing to- the decreasing of pro oxidant HM activity, puts obstacles in the development of pathological mitosis, ensures the decreasing of mutagenesis activity of the metal line mixture, that is the implementation of such therapy scheme can suspend mutagenesis in the organism.

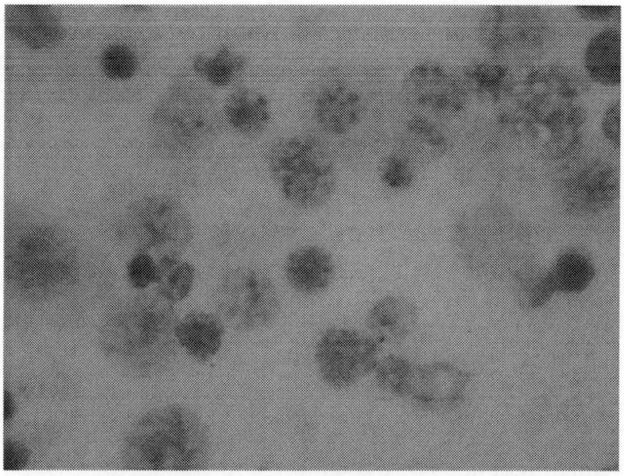

Figure 3. Cages of a red marrow of rats after treatment. Normal metaphase plates, a high mitotic index.

CONCLUSION

All unfavorable factors of the environment provoked immediate response from the liver's mono oxygenize detoxification system, one of the basic protection system, formed in the organism of the mammals with the mission of protection of its inner medium from external aggression. Failure or inability of this system to resist the external aggression leads to the contamination of the organism's inner medium, the origin of the intoxication consequence of it is the increase of acute and chronic poisonings taking one of the first places among the mortality reasons nowadays. The special place among different xenobiotic is occupied by heavy metals and their compounds possessing the ability to be accumulated in the organisms and with a very prolonged semi period of withdrawing. In under dose heavy metals exert non-specific influence which occurs through symptom less accumulation of changes in tissues and organs [10;18]. At the initial stage HM influence results in the damage of the cells elementary structure and disturbance of their functions, however the mechanisms of their toxic effect are different. As the toxicant's effect is accompanied by the change of homeostasis reception of pathogenic information is carried out by the cell through its cell membrane in the first instance. After their bioaccumulation the frustration of the organism's adaptive protection mechanisms takes place. Necessity in inactivation of these compounds leads to typical displacement in P450 cytochrome dependable metabolism of xenobiotic in liver consisting in decreasing of P450 cytochrome content in microsomal fraction and corresponding reduction of the substance oxidation level. Under pathological condition there is some reversible correlation in microsomal fraction between P450 cytochrome content and POL product concentration. Our experiments show that POL product accumulation and decreasing of activity of antioxidant system is accompanied by total reduction of the system- P450 cytochrome. In their turn the products of free- radical reactions provoked the damage of DNA molecules in the cells which is the main reason for spontaneous and induced mutagenesis [16]. As appears from the above obtained results entering of heavy metal compounds results in POL activation and exhausting of antioxidant system revealing the increased MDA level and decreased cataloes and AOA activity. The activation of POL promotes membrane destabilization and change of membrane destabilization and change of membrane- binned enzymes including oxygenize. As a result the locking of the vicious circle takes place. The tension in bio-transformative processes in liver creates the necessary prerequisites for frustration of compensatory detoxicative mechanisms of the liver and formation of pathological processes. The further entering of the toxicant provocations aggravation of the situation and it is impossible already for the natural system of organism's protection to cope with it without assistance. The obtained results showed that the incorporation of the heavy metal mixture under investigation resulted in disturbance of cell reproduction and hence led to frustration of their physiological and reparative regeneration. The damage of mitotic apparatus and blockage of cell-division in metaphase should be considered the basic peculiar feature.

The obtained results are in coincidence with the other investigators' data believing that the products of free-radical reactions, provocations the damage of DNA molecules in cells are the original causes or initial stage of the induced mutagenesis activation. To correct the exposed disturbances we used a number of means including antioxidant and entero-sorbent preparations ensuring fast removal of toxic metal line mixture from the organisms and blockage the lipoperoxidation process at the expense of increasing of the organism's antioxidant status. Great members of complexion compounds are known to remove heavy metals from the organism. However some of them taking an active part in extraction of metals-toxicants often provoked undesirable accessory phenomena- organism's impoverish in microelements. Pectin's complexion compounds of vegetable origin form resistant compounds with metals. For all this they aren't absorbed in intestine, ensuring termination of entero-hepatocellular circulation of toxic substances and products of hepatocyte destruction. The combination of marked detoxification influence of pectin together with antioxidant activity of Hepamal led to regression of pathological process which is confirmed by decreased amount of pathological mitosis. Thus the suggested tactics secures the correction of mutagenic activity of heavy metals.

REFERENCES

[1] K.V. Azarin. Heavy metals as eco-toxicants and generators of oxidative stress. News of Russian military-medicine academy. – 2008. №3 (23), app. 2. 'Environment and human health': Materials of the Sec. *S.-Peter. Int. Forum,* 1-4 July 2008.- p.62-63.

[2] A. R. Gutnikova, K.O. Makhmudov, B.A. Saidkhanov et al. On the problem of membrane-acting effect of heavy metal salts and the main correction ways. (*Russian Toxicological Reports.* – 2009. № 3. P.21-26).

[3] T.D. Degtyareva, B.A. Ratsnelson, F.A. Minigalieva et al. Biological prophylaxis of combined effect of toxic metals and organic substances. (*Russian Hygiene and sanitation.* -2007. №3. P. 37-40).

[4] N.K. Dyousembaeva, Y.A. Kulkybaev, Z. I. Namazbaeva et al. Genetic status of the population living under soil contamination with heavy metals. (*Russian Medicine of labor and industry Ecology.* 2004. №11. p. 41-43).

[5] A. H. Kasymov, A.R. Gutnikova, B.A. Saidkhanov et. al. Antioxidant efficiency of Hepamal phyto- preparation under toxic effect of the combination of metals – contaminants of environment. (*Russian Toxicological Reports.* 2008. №4. P.17-21).

[6] B.A. Katsnelson, L.F. Privalova, T.D. Degtyareva et al. Correction of some indexes of Kidney function among children subjecting to ecologically depended exposition towards lead and cadmium, as a result of implementation of the complex of antitoxic biopreparations. (*Russian Toxicological Reports;* 2007. №6. P.11-15).

[7] Korchina T. Ja. A maintenance of heavy metals in hair of children of the north of the Tyumen region. (*Russian. Hygiene and sanitation.* - 2007. № 4.-S.27-29)

[8] Kuznetsova E.A. Accumulation of heavy metals in grain crops and a way of decrease in their maintenance (*Russian. Hygiene and sanitation.* - 2007. № 4.-S.50-53)

[9] S.Y. Makhneva. Induced cytogenetic anomalies – indicators of air pollution. Ecological monitoring of forest ecosystems: all-Russian deliberation, Petrozavodsk. *Theses of reports.* Petrozavodsk. 1999. P.51.

[10] M.A. Mukasheva. Accumulation of heavy metals in biosubstrates of works of mining enterprises and population of the nearest districts.(*Russian Medicine of labor and industrial ecology.* 2004. №11. P.38-40.)

[11] V.V. Petrov., P.P. Podosinovikova, L.Y. Kubazskaya., V.B. Dolgo-Saburov. Contribution of prooxidant component in the toxic mechanisms of heavy metals and manganese. *Toxicological New.* 2004. №1. P.12-15.

[12] K.L. Sadykov. Cell and cytogenic evaluation of manganese containing dust in experimental conditions. (*Russian Medicine of labor and industrial ecology.* 2008. №2. p.18-22).

[13] L.D. Sheiko., V.P. Mamina, S.L. Balerin. Possible use of beta-carotene as a medical-preventive means. (*Russian 'Reproductive problems' Magazine.* 2001. №6.)

[14] N.L. Shushkevich. Cytogenetic non-stability during long influence of lead on the organisms of workers in lead industries. (Russian. Medicine of labor and industry. *Ecology.* 2007. №8. P.10-14).

[15] L.M. Trakhtenberg., V.S. Kolesnikov, V.P. Lukovenko. Heavy metals in environment. – (Belorussia. Minsk: "*Science and Technologies'.* 1994. P.285.)

[16] Vladimtseva T.M., Uspenskaja J.A., Nefedov V. V, Egorova A.B. Mutagenez, an induction of cellular destruction and oxidizing stress at a zinc intoxication. (*Russian. Hygiene and sanitation.* - 2002. №4.-C.56-57)

[17] Aiyar J., Bercovits H.J., Floyd R.A. et al. Reaction of chromium with glutatione or with hydrogen peroxide: identification of reactive intermediates and their role in chromium-induced DNA-damage// *Env. Health Perspect.*- 1991.- vol.92.-P. 53-62.

[18] Bashkirova J.V., Safonova N.G., Kazarinova N.V., Kolpakov M.A. Correction of intestinal biocenosis by composite mixes of sorbents and herbs ether oils at the experimental hepatitis//*Internationaler medizinischer congress.* -Hannover, 1-2 juni 2007.- P.10-11

[19] Ford. C., Hamerton Y. In the book: Evaluation of mutagenic activity of new medicines: *Methodical recommendations.* M. 1994. P. 20.

[20] Pandey J., Pandey R., Shubhashish K. Air-Borne Heavy Metal Contamination to Dietary Vegetables: A Case Study from India // *Bulletin of Environmental Contamination and Toxicology.*- 2009.- V. 83, № 6.- P. 931-936.

In: Xenobiotics: New Research
Editors: Saul F. Castaneda and Mauro L. Emerson

ISBN: 978-1-61942-616-0

Chapter 6

PHYTOREMEDIATION: AN OPTION FOR REMOVAL OF ORGANIC XENOBIOTICS FROM WATER

Ana Dordio[1,2]* *and A. J. Palace Carvalho*[1,3]
[1]Department of Chemistry, University of Évora, Évora, Portugal
[2]Institute of Marine Research, University of Évora, Évora, Portugal
[3]Centro de Química de Évora, University of Évora, Évora, Portugal

ABSTRACT

Pollution by persistent organic pollutants (pesticides, pharmaceuticals, petroleum hydrocarbons, PAHs, PCBs, etc.) is an environmental problem that is recognized worldwide. In order to address this problem, cost effective technologies have been developed and evaluated for the decontamination of soil and water resources. Phytoremediation is a promising technology that uses plants and the associated rhizosphere microorganisms to remove, transform/detoxify, or accumulate organic and inorganic pollutants present in soils, sediments, surface or ground water, wastewater, and even the atmosphere. In fact, as a result of their sedentary nature, plants have evolved diverse abilities for dealing with toxic compounds in their environment. They, therefore, possess a variety of pollutant attenuation mechanisms that makes their use in remediating contaminated land and water more feasible than physical and chemical remediation. Currently, phytoremediation is used for treating many classes of organic xenobiotics including petroleum hydrocarbons, chlorinated solvents, polycyclic aromatic hydrocarbons, pesticides, explosives, pharmaceutical compounds and their metabolites, and it involves several decontamination mechanisms. There are several different types of phytotechnologies such as, for instance, treatment constructed wetlands. The aim of this work is to present a review on the application of phytoremediation technologies for water decontamination from persistent organic pollutants, with special emphasis focused on the removal of a class of emergent pollutants that has recently been receiving a lot of attention, the pharmaceutically active compounds. Within the realm of phytotechnologies, constructed wetlands for wastewater treatment deserve a special focus as these systems have been used with success for the removal of several different types of organic xenobiotics.

* Tel: +351 - 266 745343; E-mail address: avbd@uevora.pt

1. INTRODUCTION

The rising life standards and demographic pressures exert stress on the water supply and on the quality of drinking water. Demand management and water and wastewater reuse may help mitigate some of this pressure. In wastewater management, new challenges are caused by new chemicals of concern, including many notably toxic substances and endocrine disrupters, which often pass through wastewater treatment plants (WWTPs) without being efficiently removed. Such substances may potentially cause serious impacts on aquatic ecosystems and human health.

Several thousands of different organic compounds are currently used in the modern society. These compounds include pesticides, organic solvents, explosives, dyes, phenols, petroleum hydrocarbons and a new class of emergent pollutants, pharmaceuticals. Many of these organic pollutants are persistent in the environment and potentially show adverse ecotoxicological effects. While some of these classes of pollutants are known to be present in the environment for a long time already and their toxic effects are well studied, awareness of the contamination of the aquatic environment by pharmaceuticals has only arisen more recently. This is due to the fact that these pollutants are found in that medium generally at very low concentration levels (μg L-1 – ng L-1), and it was not until the last decade that analytical methodologies and instrumentation have become available with sufficiently low detection and quantification limits to allow for the environmental monitoring of these substances (Fent et al., 2006; Petrovic and Barceló, 2007; Aga, 2008; Barceló and Petrovic, 2008; Miège et al., 2009; Bolong et al., 2009; Kümmerer, 2009). The ecotoxicity associated with this class of pollutants is also largely unassessed but potential for chronic effects caused by long term exposure and for cumulative and even synergistic action exists (Fent et al., 2006; Kim et al., 2007; Zounkova et al., 2007; Farré et al., 2008; Cooper et al., 2008; Bolong et al., 2009). Nonetheless, increasing amounts of pharmacologically active substances are consumed yearly in human and veterinary medicine which are essential for the diagnosis, treatment, or prevention of diseases.

Through excretion or disposal of unused or expired products, pharmaceuticals and their metabolites are continuously introduced into the sewage system. As many of these compounds receive inefficient treatment in WWTPs (which were not designed to deal with this type of pollutant), they eventually are released into the environment. This is considered to be the main route for contamination of the aquatic environment by pharmaceuticals (Nikolaou et al., 2007; Aga, 2008; Kasprzyk-Hordern et al., 2009; Kümmerer, 2009). Over the last years, in numerous monitoring studies, residues of lipid regulating drugs, analgesics and anti-inflammatory drugs, antibiotics, hormones, antidiabetics, neuroactive compounds and beta-blocker drugs have all been detected worldwide in wastewaters, surface waters, ground waters and even drinking waters (Fent et al., 2006; Aga, 2008; Barceló and Petrovic, 2008; Miège et al., 2009; Kümmerer, 2009).

The foreseeable environmental consequences of high environmental loads of pharmaceuticals points to the urgent need for finding ways to retain and remove these pollutants from wastewaters before they reach the receiving water bodies. Optimization of the conventional WWTP processes has been attempted by increasing hydraulic and solid retention times (Tauxe-Wuersch et al., 2005; Maurer et al., 2007; Vieno et al., 2007; Aga, 2008; Zhang et al., 2008; Miège et al., 2009). In addition, some advanced technologies have been evaluated for their capability to decontaminate waters polluted with pharmaceuticals. However, despite the sometimes high removal efficiencies attained, these processes are generally not cost-effective on a large scale (Fent et al., 2006). In fact, there is still a great need for finding applicable technologies with higher efficiencies at reasonable cost of operation and maintenance.

A phytoremediation technology for wastewater treatment that has been gaining increasing popularity over the last decades, known as constructed wetlands systems (CWS), exploits the well-known ability of natural wetlands to depurate water and attempts to optimize the processes responsible for this depuration. These systems are becoming an alternative to conventional wastewater treatment processes or are being integrated in WWTPs as a secondary or tertiary treatment step. Low cost and low maintenance are some of their most attractive characteristics (Kadlec and Wallace, 2009).

CWS may be considered, nowadays, a more mature technology for the removal of bulk pollutants such as suspended solids, organic matter, pathogens and nutrients (Vymazal et al., 1998; Kadlec and Wallace, 2009; Vymazal, 2009). Meanwhile, focus is now moving towards the removal of more specific and recalcitrant compounds for which the conventional wastewater treatment systems are not effective. In fact, CWS are currently being used more frequently for the cleanup of specific pollutant types such as organic xenobiotics and new challenges have been emerging such as the removal of pharmaceuticals and other micropollutants which present new environmental problems to be solved.

2. Persistent Organic Pollutants

The fast growth in chemical and agrochemical industries during the last century have resulted in the release of a large number of new chemical compounds into the environment. In fact, a lot of different organic compounds are now used in the day-to-day life of human beings and many of these are frequently being detected in numerous environmental monitoring studies (Ballschmiter, 1992; Daughton and Ternes, 1999; Jones and de Voogt, 1999; Gavrilescu, 2005; Doble and Kumar, 2005; Fent et al., 2006; Petrovic and Barceló, 2007; Aga, 2008; Barceló and Petrovic, 2008; Corcoran et al., 2010; Lofrano et al., 2010; El Shahawi et al., 2010; Perelo, 2010).

Over the last decades, there has been an increasing focus on a subset of harmful organic chemicals, mostly xenobiotics (synthetic compounds of anthropogenic origin that do not exist naturally in biological systems), commonly classified as Persistent Organic Pollutants (POPs) (Jones and de Voogt, 1999; Gavrilescu, 2005; El Shahawi et al., 2010). POPs are chemical substances that persist in the environment, bioaccumulate throughout the food chain, and pose a risk of causing adverse effects to human health and the environment because, when found at levels higher than background, can be toxic to biotic communities (Jones and de Voogt, 1999; El Shahawi et al., 2010). These POPs include polycyclic aromatic hydrocarbons, petroleum hydrocarbons, chlorinated solvents, explosives, dyes, phenols and pesticides (Jones and de Voogt, 1999; Gavrilescu, 2005; El Shahawi et al., 2010).

Recent advances in analytical techniques and the use of advanced instrumentation (which significantly lowered the detection and quantification limits for analyses of organic compounds in complex environmental matrices) have aided in detecting low levels of other toxic organics in the environment which came to be known as the class of emerging pollutants. An ever growing list of compounds has been detected over the last decade in raw and treated wastewater, biosolids and sediments, receiving waters, ground water and drinking water. Among these substances, pharmaceuticals have become one of the most important subset of compounds in the class of emerging pollutants (Aga, 2008; Miège et al., 2009; Kümmerer, 2009; El Shahawi et al., 2010).

Distributed into different parts of the environment, organic xenobiotics can be transported over long or short distances and can also undergo a variety of reactions and transformations (El Shahawi et al., 2010). Because of these many competing interactions the fate of such pollutants is not easy to predict and, in many cases, their ecotoxicological effects are difficult to assess (El Shahawi et al., 2010). Nevertheless, the established possibility of long-range transport of these substances to regions where they have never been used or produced and the consequent threats they may pose to the environment of the whole globe, has motivated the international community to call, at several occasions, for urgent global actions to be taken with the aim of reducing the release of these chemicals.

Pollution of soils and surface or ground waters occurs as a result of wastewater point sources, improper use and disposal or accidental release of organic chemicals into the environment. In recent years, numerous strategies and technologies have been developed for wastewater treatment or remediation of contaminated areas.

Some advanced wastewater treatment technologies that have been evaluated for the removal of POPs include advanced oxidative processes, activated carbon adsorption, membrane filtration and membrane bioreactors (Fent et al., 2006; Radjenovic et al., 2007; Kim et al., 2007; Esplugas et al., 2007; Snyder et al., 2007; Aga, 2008; Benner et al., 2008). In overall, several techniques have been developed and used for the decontamination of soils and natural waters. Some in situ processes include washing with detergent; extraction of topsoil using vacuum, steam, or hot air stripping; flooding (raising low density hydrophobic liquids to the surface above the water table); etc. Ex situ techniques include excavating the contaminated soil or pumping liquid and subjecting it to chemical oxidation, solvent extraction, adsorption, thermal desorption, etc., and later returning the treated soil or liquid back to its original place (Susarla et al., 2002; Doble and Kumar, 2005; Gan et al., 2009).

Despite the sometimes high removal efficiencies attained, these processes are not, however, widely used mainly for reasons of cost effectiveness (Zodrow, 1999; Susarla et al., 2002; Doble and Kumar, 2005; Fent et al., 2006; Gan et al., 2009). Consequently, there is a growing need for alternative treatment processes for removing POPs from soils, natural waters and wastewaters that have higher efficiencies at reasonable costs of operation/maintenance.

Phytotechnologies have been successfully used for removal of many POPs from contaminated soils, waters and wastewaters (Salt et al., 1998; Macek et al., 2000; Dietz and Schnoor, 2001; Susarla et al., 2002; Haberl et al., 2003; Pilon-Smits, 2005; Eapen et al., 2007; Olette et al., 2008; Imfeld et al., 2009; Gan et al., 2009; Aken et al., 2009). This type of approach attempts to exploit the ability of plants to adsorb, uptake and concentrate or metabolize organic xenobiotics, as well as to release root exudates that enhance compound biotransformation and microbial degradation. In particular for the removal of organic xenobiotics from raw wastewaters and WWTPs effluents, the implementation of some phytotechnologies such as constructed wetlands systems (CWS) has become a popular option (Haberl et al., 2003; Olette et al., 2008; Imfeld et al., 2009). These systems are increasingly being used to provide a form of secondary or tertiary treatment for wastewaters, and have already been used with success to remove from contaminated waters several POPs of various classes of pollutants (Williams, 2002; Haberl et al., 2003; Grove and Stein, 2005; Imfeld et al., 2009), among which some of the most important ones are briefly described below:

a) Polycyclic Aromatic Hydrocarbons

Polycyclic aromatic hydrocarbons (PAHs) consist of a large group of several hundred organic compounds characterized by containing two or more fused aromatic rings. These compounds are important pollutants because of their ubiquitous presence in the environment and the fact that some of them are considered as dangerous substances due to their toxic and mutagenic or carcinogenic potential (Kadlec and Wallace, 2009; Haritash and Kaushik, 2009; Perelo, 2010). For this reason, several of these which are considered especially harmful are included in the European Union and United States Environmental Protection Agency (EPA) priority pollutant list (Parrish et al., 2004; Gan et al., 2009; Perelo, 2010).

Both natural and anthropogenic sources contribute PAHs to the environment. Those compounds are formed during the incomplete combustion of almost any organic material (combustion of fossil fuels, forest fires, volcanic activities, automobile exhausts, etc.) but other sources are their synthesis by microorganisms, fungi, plants, and animals. Crude oil and other petroleum based products also contribute significant amounts of PAHs to the environment (Haritash and Kaushik, 2009; Gan et al., 2009).

The hazards associated with the PAHs can be overcome by the use of conventional methods which involve removal, alteration, or isolation of the pollutant. Such techniques involve excavation of contaminated soil and its incineration or containment, thermal desorption, solvent extraction or chemical oxidation. These technologies are expensive, and in many cases transfer the pollutant from one phase to another (Haritash and Kaushik, 2009; Gan et al., 2009). Phytotechnologies have been successfully used for removal of PAHs from contaminated soils, waters and wastewaters (Salt et al., 1998; Susarla et al., 2002; Parrish et al., 2004; Pilon-Smits, 2005; Eapen et al., 2007; Kadlec and Wallace, 2009; Gan et al., 2009; Sun et al., 2010; Perelo, 2010). Main mechanisms of removal should involve rhizodegradation as some PAHs are hardly taken up by plants as a result of their physicochemical characteristics (e.g. water solubility) and, thus, appear less suitable for phytodegradation (Macek et al., 2000; USEPA, 2000; Susarla et al., 2002; Newman and Reynolds, 2004; Imfeld et al., 2009; Vymazal, 2009; Fountoulakis et al., 2009).

b) Petroleum Hydrocarbons

Crude oil is a lipophilic mixture that consists of more than 17000 organic compounds and is regarded as the most complex, naturally occurring mixture of organic substances. It mainly consists of alkanes, cycloalkanes, and PAHs. Contamination of the environment by total petroleum hydrocarbons (TPHs) arises from natural as well as anthropogenic sources and is potentiated by the widespread use of so many petroleum-based products in the modern society. Human-mediated sources of TPHs include offshore oil production, marine transportation, atmospheric or aerial depositions from combustion of coal and gas flaring, direct ocean dumping, coastal, municipal and industrial wastes, and runoff (Knight et al., 1999; Doble and Kumar, 2005).

Only a relatively small number of TPHs is well characterized for toxicity. The health effects of some fractions can be well characterized based on their components or representative compounds, for example the fraction of light aromatics and, in particular, the BTEX (benzene, toluene, ethylbenzene, and xylenes) fraction. These monoaromatic hydrocarbons, which are typical constituents of TPHs wastewaters, are commonly found in some petroleum-based fuels. Of all of the BTEX compounds, benzene is of most concern, because it is the most toxic and a well-known human carcinogen. The benzene ring is a chemical structure that is very common in nature, which together with its high thermodynamic stability, provides for a significant persistence in the environment; therefore, many aromatic compounds are major environmental pollutants. Benzene contamination is, thus, a significant problem. This hydrocarbon is very soluble and mobile, especially in ground and surface waters and it is poorly biodegraded in the absence of oxygen.

Decontamination of soils and waters polluted with TPHs has been attempted by techniques involving soil solidification (binding hydrocarbon to soil), flooding, excavation of contaminated soil and subjecting it to incineration or chemical oxidation, washing with detergent, solvent extraction, adsorption, etc.. However, once again, these solutions for decontamination of polluted sites are generally expensive. Phytotechnologies for remediation of soils and natural waters has become a low-cost alternative to the conventional approaches that is been increasingly used in the latest years (USEPA, 2000; Susarla et al., 2002; Newman and Reynolds, 2004; Pilon-Smits, 2005; Eapen et al., 2007; Weishaar et al., 2009; Perelo, 2010). In particular, the application of CWS for the treatment of wastewater contaminated with TPHs has been seen as an alternative solution that has been revealed frequently effective (Vymazal et al., 1998; Knight et al., 1999; Omari et al., 2003; Gessner et al., 2005; Kadlec and Wallace, 2009; Imfeld et al., 2009; Vymazal, 2009).

c) Chlorinated Solvents

The term chlorinated solvents refers to a family of organics containing one or more chlorine atoms, which include derivatives of methane, ethane, and ethene but also polychlorinated biphenyls (PCBs). Common uses of chlorinated solvents include dry cleaning, degreasing operations, polymer manufacturing and as a chemical intermediate (Susarla et al., 2002; USEPA, 2004; Amon et al., 2007; Aken et al., 2009; Perelo, 2010).

Trichloroethylene (TCE), perchloroethylene (PCE) and polychlorinated biphenyls (PCBs) are among the most predominant chlorinated solvents which are present in the environment as contaminants (Bourg et al., 1992; Susarla et al., 2002; USEPA, 2004; Amon et al., 2007; Perelo, 2010). TCE, mainly used as a metal cleaning agent and in specialty adhesives, is a probable carcinogen and can affect kidneys, liver, lungs, and heart rate. PCE, which is also used as a metal cleaning agent and in dry cleaning, on the other hand is not classified as a carcinogen but has been known to affect the central nervous system and to cause irritation of the skin, eyes, and upper respiratory system (USEPA, 2004). PCBs are synthetic oils that do not readily react at room temperature and are primarily used as coolants and/or insulators. They are classified as probable carcinogens by the EPA and the International Agency for Research on Cancer. PCB contamination is an ecological concern, because some by-products from burning them at low temperatures (e.g. dioxins) are highly toxic and carcinogenic (USEPA, 2004; Perelo, 2010).

Most chlorinated solvents are only slightly soluble in water and, with the exception of vinyl chloride, have densities greater than that of water. This combination leads to the formation of dense non-aqueous phase liquid deposits which act as a slow releasing, continuous source of chlorinated solvents (Amon et al., 2007). For this reason they tend to remain in the environment for long periods of time and take a long time to remediate. Traditional methods for remediating chlorinated solvent contamination include natural attenuation, soil vapor extraction, air sparging and pump and treat approaches (USEPA, 2004; Amon et al., 2007). Phytoremediation mechanisms that have been successful in containing and/or remediating chlorinated solvents include rhizodegradation, phytodegradation, phytovolatilization and hydraulic control using hybrid poplar and willow trees (Salt et al., 1998; Macek et al., 2000; USEPA, 2000; Susarla et al., 2002; Newman and Reynolds, 2004; Pilon-Smits, 2005; Eapen et al., 2007; Aken et al., 2009). In the treatment of this class of POPs, the use of CWS has also revealed to be an efficient low-cost solution in several studies (Haberl et al., 2003; Amon et al., 2007; Kadlec and Wallace, 2009; Imfeld et al., 2009; Vymazal, 2009).

d) Explosives

There are three main classes of explosives: nitroaromatics, nitramines and nitrate esters. The contamination of the environment by explosives, especially by nitroesters and nitroaromatics, is a worldwide environmental problem. Contamination of soil and waters with explosives is largely due to manufacturing, storage, testing and inappropriate waste disposal of explosive chemicals and, therefore, most contaminated sites are located at ammunition factories and other places where these compounds were handled. This involved open detonation and burning of explosives at army depots, evaluation facilities, artillery ranges, and ordnance disposal sites (Hannink et al., 2002).

The primary explosives at hazardous waste sites are 2,4,6-trinitrotoluene (TNT), hexahydro-1,3,5-trinitro-1,3,5-triazine (Royal Demolition eXplosive-RDX) and octahydro-1,3,5,7-tetranitro-1,3,5,7-tetrazine (High Melting eXplosive-HMX). TNT and RDX are listed as “priority pollutants” and “possible human carcinogens” by the U.S. Environmental Protection Agency (EPA) (Etnier, 1989; Hannink et al., 2002; Van Aken, 2009). TNT is a nitroaromatic constituent of many explosives. In a refined form, TNT is stable and can be stored over long periods of time. It is relatively insensitive to blows or friction. It is readily acted upon by alkalis to form unstable compounds that are very sensitive to heat and impact. Health effects due to exposure to TNT include anemia, abnormal liver function, skin irritation, and cataracts (Hannink et al., 2002; USEPA, 2004; Van Aken, 2009). RDX is a nitramine widely used as an explosive and as a constituent in plastic explosives. RDX can cause seizures when large amounts are inhaled or eaten (Etnier, 1989; Hannink et al., 2002; USEPA, 2004). Long-term health effects on the nervous system due to low-level exposure to RDX are not known. HMX is a nitramine that explodes violently at high temperatures. It is used in nuclear devices, plastic explosives and rocket fuels. Insufficient studies on the effects of HMX to the health of humans and animals have been performed (USEPA, 2004).

Incineration, landfilling and pump and treat systems are traditional methods applied to remove explosives contamination from soil and groundwater (Hannink et al., 2002; USEPA, 2004; Van Aken, 2009). These approaches are expensive and can cause air pollution with ash generation (Susarla et al., 2002; Van Aken, 2009). Phytoremediation mechanisms that have been successful in containing and/or remediating explosives contamination include phytoextraction, phytodegradation and phytostabilization using different type of plants in constructed wetlands (Salt et al., 1998; Macek et al., 2000; USEPA, 2000; Hannink et al., 2002; Susarla et al., 2002; Newman and Reynolds, 2004; Pilon-Smits, 2005; Eapen et al., 2007; Kadlec and Wallace, 2009; Imfeld et al., 2009; Vymazal, 2009; Van Aken, 2009).

Axenic studies have shown that plants are capable of transforming TNT without microbial contribution, but very little accumulation of TNT has been found in plant material (Hughes et al., 1996; Vanderford et al., 1997; Susarla et al., 2002). Therefore, plant-enhanced degradation, or phytoremediation, of TNT by aquatic macrophytes has been proposed as a promising groundwater treatment process (USEPA, 2000).

e) Pesticides

Heavy usage of pesticides over the years (mostly via direct land application) has resulted in their ubiquitous dispersal, most typically in aquatic environments (Chaudhry et al., 2002). The intensive use of pesticides has been a public concern for decades owing to their potential risk to human health and the environment.

Pesticides can enter the water bodies via diffuse sources or via point sources. Diffuse source pesticide inputs result from field applications of pesticides and can arise not only from agricultural practices but also from some non-agricultural practices as well, affecting both surface and ground waters. These include tile drain overflow, baseflow seepage, surface and subsurface runoff, erosion, spray drift, deposition after volatilization, leaching through the soils and infiltration through river banks and beds (Reichenberger et al., 2007). Major point sources of pesticides and their treatment-resistant metabolites are WWTP effluents, farmyard runoff (either directly into streams or into the sewer system) and accidental spills (Gerecke et al., 2002; Neumann et al., 2002; Bailey et al., 2005; Gomez et al., 2007; Reichenberger et al., 2007).

Mitigation of pesticide contamination inputs into water bodies includes both the reduction of diffuse source and of point source inputs, and remediation of contaminated areas. Traditional methods of pesticide soil remediation include excavation and/or chemical oxidation processes (i.e. photocatalysis, ozonation, iron-catalyzed Fenton's reaction) or thermal processes (i.e. low temperature thermal desorption, incineration).

Phytotechnologies have been increasingly used over the latest years to remediate the more persistent pesticides (Salt et al., 1998; Macek et al., 2000; USEPA, 2000; Chaudhry et al., 2002; Susarla et al., 2002; Newman and Reynolds, 2004; Pilon-Smits, 2005; Xia and Ma, 2006; Bouldin et al., 2006; Eapen et al., 2007; Henderson et al., 2007; Olette et al., 2008; Dosnon-Olette et al., 2009). Difficulties remain, including the potential phytotoxicity of some compounds (i.e. herbicides) that were originally developed to destroy plant material. Typically the mechanisms involved in pesticide phytoremediation are phytodegradation, rhizodegradation, and phytovolatilization.

Constructed wetlands are gaining recognition as potential best management practices for the reduction of pesticide concentrations in agricultural runoffs (Schulz, 2004). Generally, their success can be attributed to their diversity of function, as they improve the potential for the range of pesticide transport and degradation processes. CWS have been applied mostly to treat wastewater from point sources such as WWTP effluents (Moore et al., 2002; Haberl et al., 2003; Braskerud and Haarstad, 2003; Ralf et al., 2003; Rose et al., 2006; Blankenberg et al., 2006; Matamoros et al., 2008b; Vymazal, 2009; Moore et al., 2009). However, field studies have shown that vegetated drainage ditches (Moore et al., 2001; Dabrowski et al., 2006) and constructed wetlands (Schulz and Peall, 2001) are also highly effective in reducing pesticide concentrations and toxicity in non-point-derived wastewaters and runoff events. As a result, vegetated agricultural water bodies have been proposed as efficient buffer zones for the protection of more sensitive receiving waters from agricultural runoffs by Moore et al. (2000).

Among the several classes of organic xenobiotics, pharmaceuticals have been attracting much attention of the international scientific community recently, although they have been contaminating many water bodies for already quite a long time (Garrison et al., 1976; Hignite and Azarnoff, 1977). The low concentrations of these compounds in the environment (typically present at trace levels, from low μg L-1 to ng L-1) associated to the unavailability, until recently, of suitably sensitive methods of analysis for these low concentration ranges, has been the main reason for the late interest on the environmental problems posed by these compounds.

Chemicals used in human and veterinary medicine are being continuously introduced in the environment, mainly due to improper disposal of unused or expired drugs, through metabolic excretion and manufacturing processes. Some of these pharmaceutical residues are discharged directly in the environment without going through appropriate treatment, but even those receiving appropriate disposal in WWTPs in many cases are not effectively removed by the conventional wastewater treatment processes (Halling-Sørensen et al., 1998; Daughton and Ternes, 1999; Heberer, 2002; Fent et al., 2006).

2.1. Pharmaceutical Compounds

Human pharmaceuticals comprise a wide ranging class of bioactive compounds with substantial variability in chemical structures, functions, behavior and activity. Their development and use aims specific biological effects and most of them are polar compounds because they are supposed to be transported within organisms through an aqueous medium. The molecular weights of the chemical molecules range typically from 200 to 1000 Da (Kümmerer, 2009).

Despite being consumed worldwide in increasing quantities, there are still not enough data available on the total use of pharmaceuticals. The consumption and application of human pharmaceuticals may vary considerably from country to country due to differences in the prevalence of diseases, treatment habits and options, or simply for market reasons. For instance, some pharmaceuticals are, in some countries, sold over the counter without prescription, while in others they are only available by prescription.

In the European Union over 3000 different pharmaceutically active substances are used in human medicine (Fent et al., 2006; Hummel et al., 2006; Ternes et al., 2007) which can be divided in several different pharmaceutical classes such as analgesics and anti-inflammatory drugs, beta-blockers, lipid regulators, neuroactive compounds and antibiotics. Many of these pharmaceuticals, from all pharmaceutical classes, are frequently detected in monitoring studies worldwide (Heberer, 2002; Fent et al., 2006; Nikolaou et al., 2007; Petrovic and Barceló, 2007; Aga, 2008; Kasprzyk-Hordern et al., 2009; Miège et al., 2009; Kümmerer, 2009).

2.1.1. Human Pharmaceuticals Sources, Fate and Effects in the Environment

In recent years, the occurrence and fate of pharmaceutical residues in the environment has gained much scientific and public attention. Over the last decade, scientists have established a large, diverse, and sometimes unexpected variety of routes through which human pharmaceuticals cross (and are distributed to) various environmental compartments. Figure 1 presents a representation of possible pathways for human pharmaceuticals in the environment.

The primary route of entry for the human pharmaceuticals, their metabolites and transformation products into the environment is through wastewater point sources (Nikolaou et al., 2007; Aga, 2008). Pharmaceuticals enter the sewage system either through excretion of non-metabolized products and their metabolites or through the use of the sewage system to dispose of excess medications. In the WWTPs these compounds generally evade efficient removal by the conventional wastewater treatment processes.

Once released into the environment via the discharge of treated wastewater, pharmaceuticals are subjected to the same potential type of transport, transfer and transformation/degradation processes as other organic contaminants. Thus, the interaction of pharmaceuticals with soil, surface and ground water is similarly complex. Transport and transformation processes of pharmaceuticals in the aquatic environment may involve sorption, hydrolysis, biological transformation/degradation, redox reactions, photodegradation, volatilization and precipitation/dissolution (Petrovic and Barceló, 2007; Aga, 2008; Kümmerer, 2008; Farré et al., 2008; Kümmerer, 2009). These processes occur continuously in the environment and influence the presence and mobility of pharmaceuticals in aquatic ecosystems. Behavior of drugs under any of these pathways for partitioning, degradation or transformation may contribute to reduce their concentrations in the environment or remove them entirely and thereby reduce their potential to impact human health and aquatic life.

Pharmaceutical compounds that are marketed in large quantities and are water soluble or slightly soluble, yet resistant to degradation through biological or chemical processes, have the greatest potential to reach steady-state levels in the environment and to be detected in surface and ground waters and in drinking water supplies (Jjemba, 2006; Petrovic and Barceló, 2007; Aga, 2008).

A major difference between pharmaceuticals and other "traditional" environmental POPs (e.g. chlorinated solvents, pesticides, PCBs, PAHs, explosives) is that pharmaceutical compounds, in general, have passed through the human digestive tract and possibly through a conventional WWTP. Two consequences of this pre-exposure to biochemical metabolism are that many drugs will enter the aquatic environment in a modified form and, on the other hand, those that are unaltered, consequently share a resistance to biotic transformation. This allows certain inferences to be made regarding the importance of various abiotic transformation processes for pharmaceutical compounds in the aquatic environment (Arnold and McNeill, 2007).

Given the water solubility of many pharmaceuticals, the abiotic processes most likely to transform them and to more permanently remove them from the aquatic environment include hydrolysis and photodegradation (Petrovic and Barceló, 2007; Aga, 2008; Kümmerer, 2008). However, considering the passage of pharmaceuticals through the digestive tract and their relatively long-residence time in aqueous environments within the WWTPs, hydrolysis reactions likely play a less important role in the aquatic fate of many pharmaceuticals that reach the environment (Arnold and McNeill, 2007). On the other hand, direct photodegradation by sunlight may be an important elimination process for pharmaceuticals with absorbances in the 290-800 nm region (Velagaleti, 1997; Andreozzi et al., 2003).

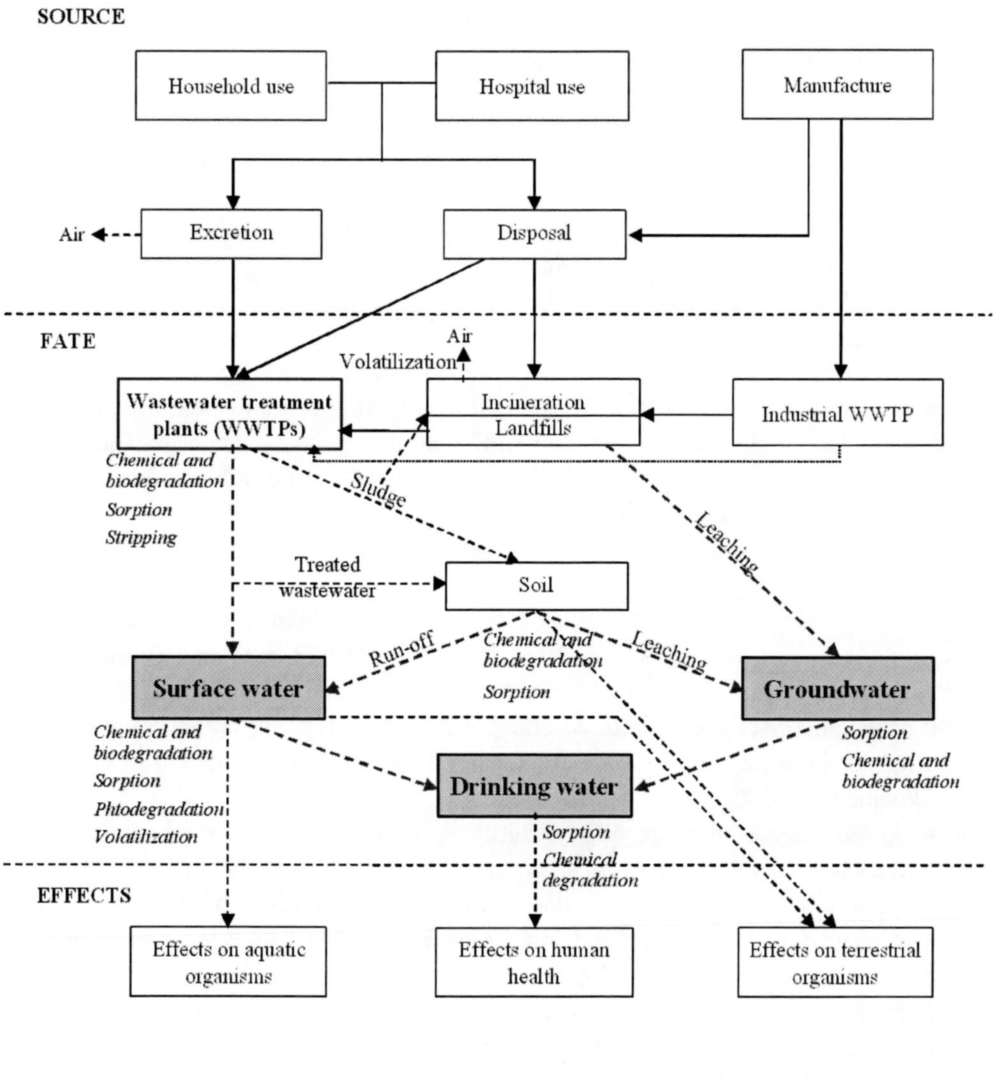

Figure 1. Pathways of human pharmaceuticals in the environment (adapted from Heberer (2002)).

In any case, the extent of the diverse abiotic and biotic processes that may potentially have an influence on the short-term behavior and long-term fate of a pharmaceutical in the environment are controlled by many factors related both with the pharmaceutical properties and with the environmental conditions. Some of the most important physical and chemical properties of the pharmaceuticals that affect their fate in the environment are the molecular structure, polarity, ionization constant, water solubility, octanol-water partition coefficient, sorption distribution coefficient and the compound's half-life.

In addition to the compound's properties, the fate of pharmaceuticals is also determined by the environmental conditions. Some of those factors include the temperature, sunlight, pH, content of organic matter in soils and sediments and redox conditions.

Evidence being accumulated over the latest years supports the case that, under ordinary conditions, pharmaceuticals have such physicochemical properties which makes them in many cases refractory to degradation and transformation and, consequently, do indeed have the potential to reach the environment (Halling-Sørensen et al., 1998; Fent et al., 2006; Nikolaou et al., 2007; Petrovic and Barceló, 2007; Aga, 2008; Kümmerer, 2009). However, little is known about the impending human or ecological hazards that can arise from the cumulative exposure to the "cocktail" of pharmaceuticals and metabolites present in the different environmental compartments (notwithstanding the low concentrations at which they are observed to occur).

Human pharmaceuticals are designed to target specific metabolic and molecular pathways and, as side-effect, when introduced in the environment they may affect analogous pathways in animals having identical or similar target organs, tissues, cells or biomolecules. Even in animals lacking or having different receptors for drugs, dissimilar modes of action may occur.

It is important to recognize that, for many drugs, their specific modes of action are not well known and often not only one but many different modes of actions occur. Therefore, the ecotoxicity of most pharmaceuticals is difficult to assess (Fent et al., 2006). In addition, the metabolites and degradation by-products of pharmaceuticals are also of concern, because many of them have a toxicity which in many cases is similar to or even higher than the parent compounds(Fent et al., 2006).

The current literature about ecotoxicological effects of human pharmaceuticals deals mainly with the short-term exposure acute toxicity evaluated in standardized tests and generally focused on aquatic organisms. Acute toxicity values are in the mg L-1 dose range for most of the pharmaceuticals detected in the environment (Halling-Sørensen et al., 1998), but reported levels in surface water are at least three orders of magnitude below (Fent et al., 2006; Nikolaou et al., 2007; Aga, 2008).

It is, on the other hand, more difficult to assess (but more relevant) whether long-term chronic effects have any environmental significance as these toxicity data is generally lacking (Fent et al., 2006). Nonetheless, some primary effects can be identified which derive from the presence of pharmaceuticals and related substances in the environment including cumulative impacts, endocrine disruption, development of antibiotic-resistant bacteria and genotoxic effects (Daughton and Ternes, 1999; Bendz et al., 2005; Fent et al., 2006; Zounkova et al., 2007; Farré et al., 2008; Fent, 2008; Cooper et al., 2008; Bolong et al., 2009).

Besides toxicity, the element of persistence is of particular importance when considering the environmental significance of pharmaceuticals. Unlike POPs like pesticides, many pharmaceuticals are not lipophilic, so they do not bioaccumulate in the environment.

However, some of those are "pseudo persistent pollutants" due to their continuous introduction in the environment. While not persistent in terms of a long half-life, these chemicals are constantly entering the environment, resulting in long-term exposure for the aquatic ecosystem.

Overall, the ecotoxicity of pharmaceuticals can be characterized as a game of risk. The possibility of negative impacts is present, and a number of researchers are trying to quantify the risk posed by various pharmaceuticals (Crane et al., 2006; Emblidge and DeLorenzo, 2006; Hernando et al., 2006b; Enick and Moore, 2007; Cooper et al., 2008; Cunningham et al., 2009).

Risk assessments rely on models that predict the physical, chemical, and biological properties and the corresponding ecotoxicity potential of non-assessed compounds by comparing them to assessed compounds. Sanderson et al. (2004) have prioritized drug classes in terms of their predicted toxicity, ranking sedatives and anti-psychotics as high priority, while anti-epileptics were ranked lower on the priority list. For specific pharmaceutical compounds Hernando et al. (2006b) and Cooper et al. (2008) calculated risk quotients from known toxicology data, and identified a set of high risk pharmaceuticals among which are ibuprofen, carbamazepine, naproxen, diclofenac and ketoprofen.

2.1.2. Human Pharmaceutical Occurrence in the Environment

The environmental occurrence of pharmaceuticals was first reported in 1976 by Garrison et al., who detected clofibric acid in treated wastewater in the USA at concentrations from 0.8 to 2 μg L−1. In Europe, the first comprehensive studies of the occurrence of pharmaceuticals in rivers and streams were reported in the mid 1980s by Watts et al. (1983), Waggott (1981), and Richardson and Bowron (1985).

In Canada, ibuprofen and naproxen were also detected in wastewaters in 1986 (Rogers et al., 1986; Nikolaou et al., 2007; Hao et al., 2007). After these findings, the occurrence of pharmaceuticals in environmental samples has been investigated in several countries: Brazil (Stumpf et al., 1999), Canada (Lishman et al., 2006; Hao et al., 2006; Comeau et al., 2008), UK (Ashton et al., 2004; Zhang and Zhou, 2007; Kasprzyk-Hordern et al., 2008), France (Andreozzi et al., 2003; Rabiet et al., 2006; Leclercq et al., 2009), Germany (Ternes, 1998; Heberer, 2002; Weigel et al., 2004; Hernando et al., 2006a; Osenbrük et al., 2007), Greece (Andreozzi et al., 2003; Koutsouba et al., 2003), Italy (Andreozzi et al., 2003; Zuccato et al., 2005), Spain (Hernando et al., 2006a; Carballa et al., 2008; Kuster et al., 2008), Sweden (Andreozzi et al., 2003; Bendz et al., 2005; Zorita et al., 2009), USA (Stackelberg et al., 2004; Benotti and Brownawell, 2007; Palmer et al., 2008; Benotti et al., 2009), among others.

The occurrence of pharmaceuticals in different environmental compartments, especially waters, has been already reviewed by several authors (Halling-Sørensen et al., 1998; Daughton and Ternes, 1999; Kümmerer, 2001; Jones et al., 2001; Heberer, 2002; Fent et al., 2006; Nikolaou et al., 2007; Petrovic and Barceló, 2007; Khetan and Collins, 2007; Aga, 2008; Kümmerer, 2008; Kümmerer, 2009). Many of the compounds that have become ubiquitous in surface waters and treated wastewater are mostly from the classes of the anti-inflammatories, antibiotics, blood lipid regulators, beta-blockers or neuroactive drugs (Nikolaou et al., 2007; Aga, 2008; Miège et al., 2009).

In all countries with developed medical care systems, some other compounds such as X-ray contrast media can also be expected to be present at appreciable concentrations in wastewaters (Heberer, 2002; Putschew and Jekel, 2007).

Among the most consumed drugs, those harder to biodegrade typically tend to be more frequently present in treated wastewaters and environmental samples. Nevertheless, the presence of some of the easily biodegradable pharmaceuticals may also still occur in effluents of WWTPs, even when removal efficiencies obtained with conventional wastewater treatment processes are high. In fact, due to heavy influent loads, some of the most consumed pharmaceuticals may, even after substantial removal during the treatment, subsist in significant amounts in the effluent that is discharged to the receiving water bodies.

The occurrence of metabolites or transformation products of pharmaceuticals has not yet been studied in much detail apart from some specific compounds (e. g. clofibric acid, 10,11-dihydro-10,11-epoxycarbamazepine, 3 – hydroxycarbamazepine, salicylic acid, hydroxyl-ibuprofen, carboxy-ibuprofen) (Farré et al., 2008; Miège et al., 2009; Leclercq et al., 2009).

2.1.3. Pharmaceutical Removal in Wastewater Treatment Plants

Recent studies have clearly shown that the removal of pharmaceutical compounds in municipal WWTPs is often incomplete. In fact, in many cases up to 90% of the initial amounts of pharmaceuticals entering the WWTPs may remain in effluent after treatment (Fent et al., 2006; Aga, 2008; Cooper et al., 2008). As a consequence, a significant fraction of the pharmaceuticals and their metabolites entering the WWTPs are discharged with the final effluent into the aquatic environment.

Conventional WWTPs were designed to remove bulk pollutants and not to deal with pharmaceuticals or other trace pollutants. Due to the highly variable physical and chemical properties of these compounds, the efficiencies by which they are removed may vary substantially. It is also mostly unknown whether WWTPs could be cost-effectively modified to reduce pharmaceutical discharges. Typically, there is very little elimination of organic micropollutants from the preliminary treatment of wastewater, and it is also unlikely that many pharmaceuticals will be removed during screening or primary sedimentation (Jones et al., 2005). As there is little biological activity, any pollutant removal at this stage will rely on both the tendency of the individual drugs to adsorb to solids and the degree of suspended solids removal in the primary sedimentation tanks (Zhang et al., 2008). Usually, there is little change in dissolved polar organics (such as pharmaceuticals) at this point, so little to no loss of polar drugs may be expected here. In general, elimination of any compound by sorption to sludge is considered relevant only when the log Kd for that compound is higher than 2.48 (i.e. Kd > 300 L kg-1) (Joss et al., 2005).

Activated sludge and trickling filters are the more common types of secondary biological treatment used in conventional WWTPs. Losses of drugs in both treatments may occur by the same mechanisms as other organic micropollutants, which include sorption to and removal in sludge and/or chemical degradation/transformation (such as hydrolysis) and biotransformation/biodegradation (aerobic, anoxic and anaerobic). In activated sludge processes, little loss by volatilization during aeration (stripping) is expected due to the low volatility of most pharmaceuticals (Larsen et al., 2004; Miège et al., 2009). In fact, it is found that Henry coefficients of over ~ 10−3 are required for significant stripping in a bioreactor with fine bubble aeration (Larsen et al., 2004).

Drugs remaining in the wastewater after primary and secondary treatment may be eliminated by tertiary or advanced treatments. Advanced treatment techniques such as chemical oxidation (e.g. ozonation) and membrane treatment (e.g. ultrafiltration) have been shown to be able to remove pharmaceuticals. How effectively they do so varies with the treatment conditions employed but, in some cases, it was possible to achieve levels below detection limits in drinking water treatment works (Ikehata et al., 2006; Esplugas et al., 2007; Guil et al., 2007). However, in most countries only a small number of WWTPs include these adaptations.

The issue of emergent pollutants such as pharmaceuticals and the need for regulating water quality parameters for this type of contamination have been raised several times by specialists (Robinson et al., 2007; Bolong et al., 2009). In fact, environmental agencies worldwide are evolving towards a greater awareness to this problem, electing these new substances as priority pollutants and requiring new environmental risk assessments to be carried out as part of the process of approving new substances for public use (Kot-Wasik et al., 2007). In this context, it is foreseeable that wastewater treatment requirements become more stringent in the coming years in terms of the limiting concentrations of many of these substances in the WWTPs effluents. To meet these new requirements, many of the existing conventional WWTPs will have to be adapted or reformed in the coming years. Consequently, there is a growing need for alternative wastewater treatment processes for removing pharmaceuticals from waters that have higher efficiencies at reasonable costs of operation/maintenance.

An alternative low-cost wastewater treatment option for removal of pharmaceuticals from wastewater may be the use of phytotechnologies such as constructed wetlands systems which have already shown high efficiencies in removing some pharmaceuticals (Matamoros et al., 2005; Matamoros et al., 2007a; Conkle et al., 2008; Matamoros et al., 2008a; Park et al., 2009; Matamoros et al., 2009a; Dordio et al., 2009a; Dordio et al., 2010) and other organic recalcitrant compounds (e.g. pesticides, poliaromatic hydrocarbons, explosives, chlorinated solvents, petroleum hydrocarbons) from contaminated waters (Haberl et al., 2003; Matamoros et al., 2007b; Matamoros et al., 2008b; Imfeld et al., 2009).

3. Phytoremediation Technologies

Phytoremediation is a broad term that has been in use since the early 1990s to refer to a group of technologies that use plants and its associated microorganisms, enzymes and water consumption to remove, retain, immobilize or transform/degrade pollutants, primarily of anthropogenic origin, from soil, sludges, sediments, water and wastewater and even the atmosphere (Salt et al., 1998; Macek et al., 2000; USEPA, 2000; Dietz and Schnoor, 2001; Susarla et al., 2002; Pilon-Smits, 2005; Vangronsveld et al., 2009). Phytoremediation is appealing because it is relatively inexpensive and aesthetically pleasing to the public, compared to alternate remediation strategies (e.g. involving excavation, or chemical in situ stabilization/conversion) (Zodrow, 1999; Macek et al., 2000; Susarla et al., 2002; Eapen et al., 2007).

Phytoremediation can be performed both in situ and ex situ. In the latest years efforts have focused on accelerating degradation of organic pollutants, usually in concert with root rhizosphere microorganisms, or remove hazardous heavy metals from soils or water (USEPA, 2000).

Several mechanisms have been identified by which plants can reduce pollutants availability in various environmental compartments. These include phytoextraction, phytovolatilization, phytodegradation, rhizodegradation, rhizofiltration, phytostabilization, and hydraulic control (Salt et al., 1998; ITRC, 1999; Macek et al., 2000; USEPA, 2000; Dietz and Schnoor, 2001; Susarla et al., 2002; Singh and Jain, 2003; Pilon-Smits, 2005):

- phytoextraction/phytoaccumulation – this process involves the removal of pollutants by the roots of plants and subsequent transport to aerial plant parts; pollutants accumulated in stems and leaves are harvested with accumulating plants and removed from the site;
- phytodegradation – this consists on the conversion of organic pollutants into compounds with reduced toxicity through the action of internal or secreted enzymes;
- phytovolatilization – through this process soluble pollutants are taken up with water by the roots, transported to the leaves and volatilized into the atmosphere through the stomata; amounts of pollutants transpired are proportional to the water flow and usually relatively low;
- rhizodegradation – breakdown of organic pollutants through microbial enzymatic activity is called rhizodegradation; the types of plants growing in the contaminated area influence the amount, diversity and activity of microbial populations;
- rhizofiltration – this mechanism of pollutants retention involves either adsorption or absorption by plants roots; consequently, large root surface areas are usually required for these processes;
- phytostabilization – through this process, accumulation by plant roots or precipitation in the soil by root exudates immobilizes and reduces the availability of soil pollutants; plants growing on polluted sites also stabilize the soil and can serve as a groundcover thereby reducing wind and water erosion and direct contact of the pollutants with animals;
- hydraulic control – containment of pollutants within a site can also be achieved by limiting the spread of a contaminant plume through plant evapotranspiration.

In the soil/water-plant-atmosphere continuum, a specific contaminant can be remediated at specific points along this continuum by different phytoremediation mechanisms. This is shown in Figure 2.

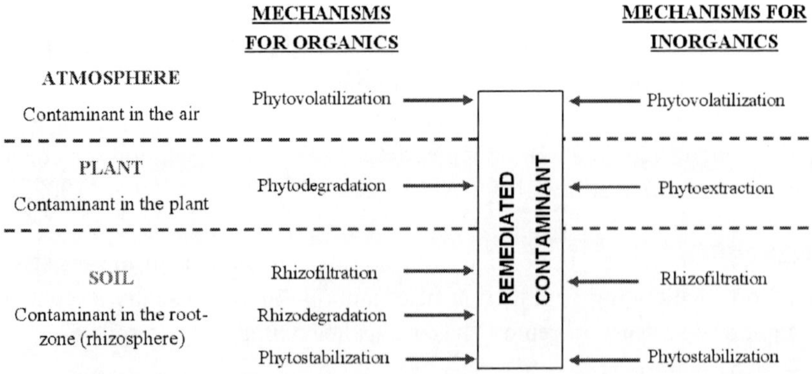

Figure 2. Contaminant fate in the Soil/Water-Plant-Atmosphere Continuum (adapted from ITRC (1999)).

As any other technology, phytoremediation has both advantages and limitations. Several benefits can be obtained from the use of phytoremediation (ITRC, 1999; Macek et al., 2000; USEPA, 2000; Pilon-Smits, 2005):

- Phytoremediation installations provide improved aesthetics and receive a better acceptance from the public as they are less invasive and destructive than other technologies. They additionally may provide habitat to animals and promote biodiversity.
- Phytoremediation is a low-cost technology compared to other treatment methods. Studies have indicated that implementing phytoremediation may result in cost savings of 50 to 80 % over traditional technologies.
- It is easy to implement and maintain, and it is effective for a variety of organic and inorganic compounds.
- It reduces the amount of dust emission and may promote better air quality in the vicinity of the site. Vegetation also helps reduce erosion by wind or water.

Phytoremediation technology, however, has its limitations and is not applicable or successful for all sites and situations. Some disadvantages must be noted (ITRC, 1999; Macek et al., 2000; USEPA, 2000; Pilon-Smits, 2005):

- Extremely high concentrations of pollutants may not allow plants to grow or cause them to die. So, phytoremediation is more effective or limited to lower concentrations of contaminants.
- For phytoremediation to be successful, contaminants must be within reach of plants roots, therefore it is restricted to sites which shallow contamination, with effective depth limited by the size of the rooting zone.
- Phytoextraction can cause contaminants to accumulate in plant tissues. The potential for ecological exposure through consumption of contaminated plants by animals and possible effect on the food chain is an environmental concern. Harvesting of contaminated biomass may be required.
- Phytovolatilization may remove contaminants from the subsurface but might then cause increased airborne exposure. In general, the fate of contaminants is often unclear, which may raise important issues with the potential for the dissemination of some pollutants in the environment.
- If non-native species are selected for phytoremediation, the consequences of introducing them in the ecosystem may be unknown or unexpected.
- Phytoremediation may take a longer time to achieve remediation goals (sometimes several year) than is required by other treatment technologies. For instance, a tree stand may take several growing seasons to be established and for contaminant concentrations to be reduced.
- The success of phytoremediation may be seasonal, depending on location. Its effectiveness may be variable, affected by climate conditions.

Several different types of phytotechnology applications can be considered in relation to the different ways the plants and their rhizosphere organisms are used. They can be used as filters in constructed wetlands or in a hydroponic setup, the latter consisting of a rhizofiltration treatment. Trees can be used as a hydraulic control barrier to create an upward water flow in the root zone, preventing contamination to leach down or to prevent a contaminated ground water plume from spreading horizontally (USEPA, 2000; Pilon-Smits, 2005). Plants can also be used to stabilize pollutants in soil, either simply by preventing erosion, leaching or runoff, or by converting pollutants to less bioavailable forms, for example through precipitation. Other uses may include phytoextraction of pollutants followed by harvesting of the aerial plant parts, and the plant material can subsequently be used for nonfood purposes (e.g. wood, cardboard) or ashed and diposed in a landfill. In the case of valuable metals, recycling of the accumulated element can be carried out, thus comprising a technology which is termed phytomining (Pilon-Smits, 2005).

In several phytotechnologies a given mechanism for the pollutant's removal may be predominant but the various possible mechanisms are not mutually exclusive. On the contrary, several mechanisms can occur simultaneously, either concurrently or cooperatively, in the case of some phytotechnologies. For instance, in a more complex phytotechnology application such as a constructed wetlands system, rhizodegradation and phytostabilization, phytoextraction, phytodegradation amd phytovolatilization can all contribute in varying degrees to the overall effect of the system on the pollutants removal.

4. Constructed Wetlands Systems

Constructed wetlands systems (CWS) are engineered systems designed and constructed to make use of the natural processes involving wetland vegetation, soil and their associated microbial assemblages to assist in wastewater treatment. The concerted action of all these components (support matrix, vegetation and microbial populations), through a variety of chemical, physical and biological processes, is responsible for the depuration of wastewaters achieved in a CWS. These systems take advantage of many of the same processes that occur in natural wetlands, but do so within a more controlled environment. CWS can be classified in several different types, as depicted in Figure 3, according to the type of water flow regime: free water surface (FWS) constructed wetlands, vertical subsurface flow (VSSF) constructed wetlands, and horizontal subsurface flow (HSSF) constructed wetlands; and according to the type of vegetation, especially in respect to the way it is anchored to the bottom of the system: CWS with free-floating plants, CWS with submerged plants, and CWS with emergent plants.

CWS have been used to treat a variety of wastewaters (municipal, industrial and agricultural) and including urban runoff (USEPA and USDA-NRCS, 1995; Cooper et al., 1996; Vymazal et al., 1998; Sundaravadivel and Vigneswaran, 2001; Haberl et al., 2003; Stottmeister et al., 2003; Scholz and Lee, 2005; Kadlec and Wallace, 2009; Vymazal, 2009).

In the past, CWS have been used mainly as wastewater treatment alternatives or complementary to the conventional treatment for domestic wastewaters of small communities. Thus, CWS have been mostly applied in the removal of bulk wastewater pollutants such as suspended solids, organic matter, excess of nutrients and pathogens.

More recently, CWS applications for dealing with more specific pollutants, such as organic xenobiotics, have been meeting a larger interest and have been the subject of an increasing number of studies.

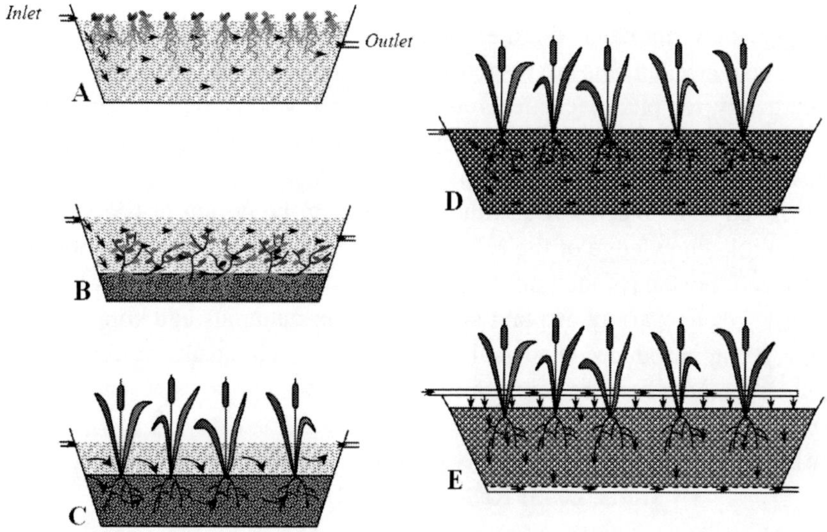

Figure 3. Different types of CWS (A, FWS with free-floating plants; B, FWS with submerged plants; C, FWS with emergent plants; D, Horizontal SSF; E, Vertical SSF) (adapted from Dordio et al. (2008)).

In many of such studies, CWS have been proving to be efficient and cost-effective solutions for the removal of some organic xenobiotics such as pesticides, azo dyes, explosives and petroleum hydrocarbons (Williams, 2002; Haberl et al., 2003; Braskerud and Haarstad, 2003; Low et al., 2008; Davies et al., 2008; Imfeld et al., 2009; Vymazal, 2009; Moore et al., 2009; Tang et al., 2009). However, their evaluation for the removal of pharmaceuticals, their metabolites and transformation products is currently a very active topic of research and can be considered as work still in progress (Gross et al., 2004; Dordio et al., 2007; Matamoros et al., 2007b; Conkle et al., 2008; Matamoros et al., 2008a; Matamoros et al., 2008b; Park et al., 2009; Matamoros et al., 2009a; Dordio et al., 2009a; Matamoros et al., 2009b; Dordio et al., 2009b; Dordio et al., 2010). Ultimately, the optimization of CWS for the removal of more specific target compounds requires a basic knowledge of the processes involved in the removal of the pollutants and the interactions between those and the CWS components. New trends in CWS research are moving towards the study of such processes and interactions and focus on the selection and optimization of the CWS components for more specific applications.

4.1. Organic Xenobiotics Removal in CWS

A specialized use of CWS for the removal of specific organic compounds or classes of compounds has been developing as a growing type of CWS applications in comparison to the treatment of bulk pollutants. Significant work exists with wastewater contaminated with organic xenobiotics from the petroleum industry, food processing industry, pesticide contaminated agricultural runoff, landfill leachates, and waters containing surfactants, solvents or mineral oils (Vymazal et al., 1998; Williams, 2002; Haberl et al., 2003; Imfeld et al., 2009; Vymazal, 2009). Very little is commonly known, about the exact pathways of the organic xenobiotics removal in CWS. Given the diversity of chemical characteristics of these compounds, which despite being classified under a common designation of xenobiotics are in fact formed by widely unrelated families of chemical substances, it is of no surprise that several very diverse mechanisms are responsible for their removal. The same observation can be made specifically for pharmaceuticals as this subset of xenobiotics is equally varied in terms of their chemical properties. A comprehensive description of organic xenobiotics removal in CWS is, thus, not an easy task to accomplish and these systems have been and still are largely operated as a "black box". Although much of the design of CWS in the past has been done with little knowledge of the roles played by each component and how its function could be optimized, nowadays the knowledge that has been accumulating is beginning to be applied. A much greater variety of plant species, matrix materials and constructed wetlands designs is now, being introduced. The goals of the target contaminants to remove in CWS are also becoming progressively more ambitious.

Table 1. Abiotic and biotic processes involved in xenobiotics removal in CWS (Pilon-Smits, 2005; Reddy and DeLaune, 2008)

Processes	Description
Abiotic	
Sorption	Including adsorption and absorption, the chemical processes occurring at the surface of plants roots and solid matrix that result in a short-term retention or long-term immobilization of xenobiotics.
Hydrolysis	The chemical breakdown of organics by the action of water, a process which is pH-dependent.
Photodegradation	Degradation of organic xenobiotics by the action of sunlight
Redox reactions	Modification, which sometimes may be quite substantial, of xenobiotics due to the action of oxidizing or reducing agents. Redox reactions are also frequently brought about by biotic agents (e.g. bacteria), or enzymatically catalyzed.
Precipitation	For those compounds which can exist in several forms with different water solubilities, the conversion into the most insoluble forms.
Filtration	Removal of particulate matter and suspended solids.
Volatilization	Release of some organic xenobiotics as vapors, which occurs when these compounds have significant vapor pressures.
Biotic	
Aerobic/anaerobic biodegradation	Metabolic processes of microorganisms, which play a significant role in organic xenobiotics removal in CWS.
Phytodegradation	Breakdown of organic xenobiotics having first been taken up by plants.
Rhizodegradation	Enhancement of microbial degradation of some organic xenobiotics by the stimulus provided by substances released in roots exudates.
Phytovolatilization	Uptake and transpiration of volatile organics through the aerial plant parts.

4.1.1. Main Removal Processes in CWS

Organic xenobiotics removal by CWS involves several interdependent processes which may be classified as abiotic (physical or chemical) or biotic (carried out by living organisms such as plants and microorganisms). These processes are basically the same occurring in natural wetlands and also identical to those responsible for the fate of xenobiotics in the environment. The way in which CWS differ from natural wetlands is that CWS are engineered systems where these processes occur in a controlled environment and conditions are optimized in order to maximize pollutants removal. The primary abiotic and biotic processes that participate in removing organic xenobiotics from contaminated water in a CWS are described in Table 1.

Removal of pollutants from water may be accomplished through storage in the wetland solid matrix and in the vegetation, or through losses to the atmosphere. A basic understanding of how these processes operate in wetlands is extremely helpful for assessing the potential applications, benefits and limitations of CWS.

a) Abiotic Processes

A wide range of physical and chemical processes are involved in the abiotic removal of contaminants in CWS. The most important abiotic removal process occurring in CWS, at the surface of plants roots and solid media, is sorption, resulting in a short-term retention or long-term immobilization of the contaminants (Vymazal et al., 1998; Reddy and DeLaune, 2008; Kadlec and Wallace, 2009). The type of materials that compose the support matrix will have a strong influence over the occurrence of sorption processes. The chemical characteristics of the solid matrix determines its capacity to sorb pollutants (Muller et al., 2007; Reddy and DeLaune, 2008b) but retention in abiotic components is also a function of several characteristics of the wastewater, such as its dissolved organic matter content, pH and electrolyte composition, as well as of the pollutant itself. In addition, a good hydraulic conductivity of the support matrix, which avoids the occurrence of overland flows and preferential channeling, is crucial for a good and uniform contact of the wastewater with the CWS media and, thus, for the efficiency of the system (Vymazal et al., 1998; Kadlec and Wallace, 2009).

Other common abiotic processes such as hydrolysis, photodegradation, redox reactions and volatilization (Table 1) can also contribute, in varied extents, to the removal of some particular classes of compounds, depending on their specific properties. However, with exception of sorption, abiotic processes are not, in general, major removal processes for most organic compounds such as pharmaceuticals because either the conditions in CWS or the properties of the compounds are not suitable. For example, photodegradation can only be significant in FWS systems, if plant density is not too high (such that it does not cause too much shade) and if the compounds are photosensitive. In SSF systems photodegradation does not occur in appreciable extent as the water level is below the solid matrix surface and, therefore, exposure of the pollutants to sunlight is very limited in this type of systems. The process of volatilization is also of modest importance for substances with low volatility, as is the case of most pharmaceuticals. Where CWS are used as a tertiary treatment stage after conventional secondary treatment in a WWTP, organic compounds do not suffer, in most cases, appreciable hydrolysis either, as they have been already subjected to such type of processes in secondary treatment stage (and, in case of pharmaceuticals, previously in the human digestive system as well). Therefore, the organic xenobiotics present in CWS influents are those that have resisted such hydrolysis processes or they are the transformation products of those substances that did not resist it.

b) Biotic Processes

CWS are biological systems in which biological processes play a major role in the removal of pollutants. The two biotic components which are responsible in CWS by the biological contribution to the removal of organics are the wetland vegetation and the microbial populations.

The plants growing in natural wetlands (often called wetland plants or macrophytes), are also typically the plant species used in constructed wetlands as these are well adapted to the water saturated conditions found in these systems (Brix, 1994; Brix, 1997; Kadlec and Wallace, 2009). Major roles of macrophytes in CWS include the filtration of large debris; provision of surface area for microorganisms development and release of exudates by roots (normally including organic acids, sugars, amino acids, vitamins and enzymes (Macek et al., 2000; Alkorta and Garbisu, 2001)) that stimulate microorganisms' growth; enhancement of the hydraulic conductivity of the support matrix (roots and rhizomes growth help to prevent clogging in the matrix); transport and release of oxygen through the roots (which increases aerobic degradation and nitrification); and attenuation of the wastewater pollutants load (nutrient and xenobiotics uptake) (Brix, 1994; Sundaravadivel and Vigneswaran, 2001; Haberl et al., 2003; Kadlec and Wallace, 2009).

In CWS, an increasingly important role is being attributed to plants in removing poorly or non-biodegradable organic xenobiotics through their capacity to sorb them in their roots and even uptake them and sequester/transform them in their tissues (Macek et al., 2000; Korte et al., 2000; Dietz and Schnoor, 2001; Pilon-Smits, 2005; Collins et al., 2006). In fact, direct uptake by plants is a widely recognized process for inorganic pollutants removal. In the case of some organic substances, plant uptake has been observed to also play a significant role among biotic processes, especially for those compounds with a moderate hydrophobicity ($0.5 < \log K_{ow} < 3.5$) (Dietz and Schnoor, 2001; Schroder and Collins, 2002; Pilon-Smits, 2005). Nevertheless, action of microorganisms is generally accepted to be the major route for organic xenobiotics elimination in wetlands. However, even in these microbial processes, plants do play a relevant role, through the influence of exudates released in the rhizosphere which have the effect of stimulating the development and the activity of microorganisms (apart from also contributing, in some cases, to the catalytic degradation of pollutants) (Macek et al., 2000; Singer et al., 2003; Pilon-Smits, 2005).

Although microorganisms may also provide a measurable amount of contaminant uptake and storage, it is their metabolic processes that play the most significant role in the decomposition of organic compounds through the transformation of complex molecules into simpler ones (Reddy and DeLaune, 2008). This provides an important biological mechanism for removal of a wide variety of organic compounds. However, the efficiency and rate of organic compounds degradation by microorganisms is highly variable for different compounds types.

The characteristics of the biotic components (vegetation and microorganisms) obviously also have a tremendous influence on the CWS behavior. Microorganisms populations develop naturally in CWS and are exposed to similar factors as those affecting their development in WWTPs. However, the characteristics of these microbial populations can be modified by inoculation of the CWS with strands that are more adequate for the purpose of the system. Important characteristics of both microorganisms and plants are their tolerance to the more toxic pollutants (at typical wastewater concentrations) and their capacity to, respectively, biodegrade or uptake them. In the case of the vegetation, other factors related with the CWS design such as plant density and layout of the specimens (e.g. the way specimens of different species may be intermixed when planted in the beds) all have to be considered and carefully planned as their influence may range from subtle differences in the system's behavior to more pronounced impacts in the overall efficiency (Kadlec and Wallace, 2009). In particular, the cycles of vegetative activity of some species in addition to variations of climate conditions may lead to significant seasonal changes in the system's efficiency, which in some cases may be mitigated by using polycultures of vegetation (Kadlec and Wallace, 2009).

4.1.2. Pharmaceutical Removal in CWS

Studies conducted so far on the removal of pharmaceuticals in CWS have shown the potential of these systems to remove a wide variety of compounds (Table 2). However, there is still ample work of optimization to be carried out on these systems, which must be based on a better understanding of how the several processes involved perform their functions and interoperate. A more profound characterization of the roles played by each CWS component in the overall pharmaceuticals removal efficiency, related with the properties of each substance involved, is also necessary to guide an optimal selection of each component. The available studies on this subject, although providing valuable information, are still scarce and further work is still necessary.

4.2. The Role of Plants in Organic Xenobiotics Removal

Plants play an important role in the biotic processes of organics removal in CWS, as described previously involving several processes of which many details still remain to be known or fully understood. Subjected to the direct or indirect action of plants, xenobiotics can be stabilized or degraded in the rhizosphere, adsorbed or accumulated in the roots and transported to the aerial parts, volatilized or degraded inside the plant tissues (Figure 4).

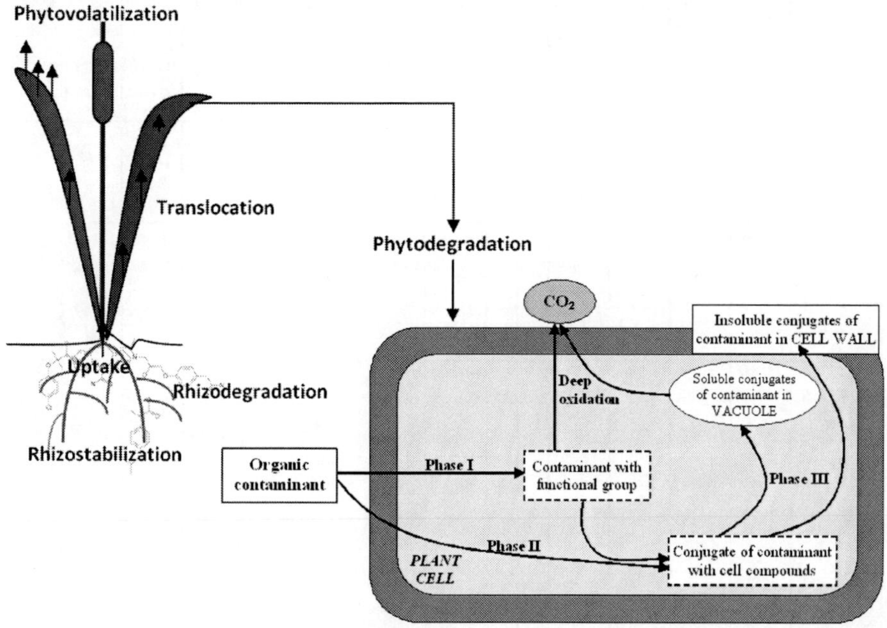

Figure 4. Major removal processes and transformation pathways of organic xenobiotics in plants (adapted from Kvesitadze et al. (2006) and Abhilash et al. (2009)).

Table 2. Pharmaceutical removal in different types of CWS

Organic compound	Physico-chemical properties			Type of CWS [c]	Type of substrate /plant [d]	% Removed [e]	Removal processes suggested by authors	References
	S_W [*, a] (25°C) (mg L^{-1})	$\log K_{ow}$ [*,b] (25° C)	pKa [*]					
Ibuprofen	21	3.97	4.9	HSSF	Gravel/ *Phragmites australis*	48 (deep) 81 (shallow)	Microbial degradation, sorption	(Matamoros et al., 2005)
				HSSF	Gravel/ *Phragmites australis*	71	ibid.	(Matamoros and Bayona, 2006)
				VSSF	Gravel/ *Phragmites australis*	99	ibid.	(Matamoros et al., 2007a)
				HSSF	Gravel/ *Phragmites australis*	52	ibid.	(Matamoros et al., 2008a)
				HSSF	n.d.	65	ibid.	(Matamoros et al., 2009a)
				VSSF	n.d.	89	ibid.	
				FWS	*Typha* spp. + *Phragmites australis*	95 (Winter) 96 (Summer)	ibid.	(Matamoros et al., 2008b)
				Lagoon + VSSF	Gravel/ *Hydrocottle* spp. + *Phragmites australis*	> 99	n. d.	(Conkle et al., 2008)
				CWS (microcosms)	Expanded clay/ *Typha* spp	82 (Winter) 96 (Summer)	Microbial degradation, plant uptake, sorption	(Dordio et al., 2010)
Carbamazepine	17.7	2.45	14	HSSF	Gravel/ *Phragmites australis*	26 (deep) 16 (shallow)	Sorption	(Matamoros et al., 2005)
				HSSF	Gravel/ *Phragmites australis*	16	ibid.	(Matamoros and Bayona, 2006)
				VSSF	Gravel/ *Phragmites australis*	26	ibid.	(Matamoros et al., 2007a)
				HSSF	Gravel/ *Phragmites australis*		ibid.	(Matamoros et al., 2008a)
				HSSF	n.d.	38	ibid.	(Matamoros et al., 2009a)

Organic compound	Physico-chemical properties			Type of CWS [c]	Type of substrate /plant [d]	% Removed [e]	Removal processes suggested by authors	References
	S_W [*, a] (25°C) (mg L^{-1})	$\log K_{ow}$ [*,b] (25° C)	pKa [*]					
				FWS	*Typha* spp. + *Phragmites australis*		ibid.	(Matamoros et al., 2008b)
				FWS	*Acorus* + *Typha* spp.	65	Plant uptake	(Park et al., 2009)
				CWS (microcosms)	Expanded clay/ *Typha* spp	88 (Winter) 97 (Summer)	Sorption, plant uptake	(Dordio et al., 2010)
Clofibric acid	583	2.57	3.18	*HSSF*	Gravel/ Phragmites australis	n.r.	-	(Matamoros et al., 2005)
				FWS	Typha spp. + Phragmites australis	32 (Winter) 36 (Summer)	n.d	(Matamoros et al., 2008b)
				CWS (microcosms)	Expanded clay/ Typha spp	48 (Winter) 75 (Summer)	Sorption, plant uptake	(Dordio et al., 2010)
Atenolol	13300	0.16	9.6	*Lagoon + VSSF*	Gravel/ Hydrocottle spp. + Phragmites australis	> 99	n.d.	(Conkle et al., 2008)
				FWS	Acorus + Typha spp.	97	n.d	(Park et al., 2009)
				CWS (microcosms)	Expanded clay/ Typha spp or Phragmites australis	> 92	Sorption, plant uptake	(Dordio et al., 2009a)
Naproxen	15.9	3.18	4.15	*HSSF*	Gravel/ Phragmites australis	85	Microbial degradation, sorption	(Matamoros and Bayona, 2006)
				VSSF	Gravel/ Phragmites australis	89	ibid.	(Matamoros et al., 2007a)
				HSSF	n.d.	45	ibid.	(Matamoros et al., 2009a)
				VSSF	n.d.	92	ibid.	
				FWS	Typha spp. + Phragmites australis	52 (Winter) 92 (Summer)	ibid.	(Matamoros et al., 2008b)
Ketoprofen	51	3.12	4.45	*HSSF*	Gravel/ Phragmites australis	38	Sorption	(Matamoros and Bayona, 2006)

Table 2. Continued

Organic compound	Physico-chemical properties			Type of CWS [c]	Type of substrate /plant [d]	% Removed [e]	Removal processes suggested by authors	References
	S_W [*, a] (25°C) (mg L^{-1})	$\log K_{ow}$ [*,b] (25° C)	pKa [*]					
				HSSF	n.d.	90	ibid.	(Matamoros et al., 2009a)
				VSSF	n.d.	n.r.	ibid.	
				FWS	Typha spp. + Phragmites australis	97 (Winter) 99 (Summer)	Photodegradation	(Matamoros et al., 2008b)
Diclofenac	2.4	4.51	4.15	*HSSF*	Gravel/ Phragmites australis	15	Sorption	(Matamoros and Bayona, 2006)
				VSSF	Gravel/ Phragmites australis	73	ibid.	(Matamoros et al., 2007a)
				HSSF	n.d.	21	ibid.	(Matamoros et al., 2009a)
				FWS	Typha spp. + Phragmites australis	73 (Winter) 96 (Summer)	ibid.	(Matamoros et al., 2008b)
Caffeine	21600	-0.07	10.4	*HSSF*	Gravel/ Phragmites australis	97	Microbial degradation, sorption	(Matamoros and Bayona, 2006)
				VSSF	Gravel/ Phragmites australis	99	ibid.	(Matamoros et al., 2007a)
				HSSF	n.d.	97	ibid.	(Matamoros et al., 2009a)
				VSSF	n.d.	99	ibid.	
				Lagoon + VSSF	Gravel/ Hydrocottle spp. + Phragmites australis	> 99	n.d.	(Conkle et al., 2008)
Salicylic acid	2240	2.26	2.97	*HSSF*	Gravel/ Phragmites australis	96	Microbial degradation, sorption	(Matamoros and Bayona, 2006)
				VSSF	Gravel/ Phragmites australis	98	ibid.	(Matamoros et al., 2007a)

Organic compound	Physico-chemical properties			Type of CWS [c]	Type of substrate /plant [d]	% Removed [e]	Removal processes suggested by authors	References
	S_W [*, a] (25°C) (mg L^{-1})	$\log K_{ow}$ [*, b] (25° C)	pKa [*]					
				HSSF	n.d.	95	ibid.	(Matamoros et al., 2009a)
Sulfamethoxazole	610	0.89		*Lagoon + VSSF*	Gravel/ Hydrocottle spp. + Phragmites australis	91	n.d.	(Conkle et al., 2008)
				FWS	Acorus + Typha spp.	30		(Park et al., 2009)
Metoprolol	16900	1.88	9.6	*Lagoon + VSSF*	Gravel/ Hydrocottle spp. + Phragmites australis	92	n.d.	(Conkle et al., 2008)
Sotalol	5510	0.24		*Lagoon + VSSF*	Gravel/ Hydrocottle spp. + Phragmites australis	30	n.d.	(Conkle et al., 2008)
Acetaminophen	14000	0.46	9.38	*Lagoon + VSSF*	Gravel/ Hydrocottle spp. + Phragmites australis	100	n.d.	(Conkle et al., 2008)
Gemfibrozil	10.9	4.77		*Lagoon + VSSF*	Gravel/ Hydrocottle spp. + Phragmites australis	64	n.d.	(Conkle et al., 2008)

[*] PHYSPROP, 2009.

[a] Sw=Water solubility.

[b] Kow=Octanol-water partition coefficient.

[c] CWS: Constructed wetlands system; HSSF: Horizontal subsurface flow; VSSF: Vertical subsurface flow; FWS: Free Water Surface.

[d] n.d.: not detailed.

[e] n.r.: not removed.

Many organic pollutants can be readily taken up by plants but, as consequence of being xenobiotic, there are no specific transporters for these compounds in the plant membranes. Therefore, they move into and within plant tissues via diffusion (or passive uptake) (Dietz and Schnoor, 2001; Pilon-Smits, 2005; Collins et al., 2006). The flux is driven by the water potential gradient created throughout the plant during transpiration, which depends on the plants characteristics and the CWS environmental conditions. Translocation of the compounds is highly dependent on their concentrations and physicochemical properties such as water solubility, log Kow and pKa (Korte et al., 2000; USEPA, 2000; Alkorta and Garbisu, 2001).

An optimal hydrophobicity may exist such that the organic compound has a tendency to bind to the lipid bilayer of the membrane but not too strongly so that transport can still occur. Direct uptake by roots is usually an efficient removal mechanism for moderately hydrophobic organic chemicals (log Kow = 0.5 – 3.5) (USEPA, 2000; Dietz and Schnoor, 2001; Pilon-Smits, 2005). In general, hydrophobic chemicals (log Kow > 3.5) are bound so strongly to the lipophilic root solids and cell walls that they cannot easily enter and be translocated in the plant. On the other hand, chemicals that are quite water soluble (log Kow < 0.5) are not sufficiently sorbed to roots nor effectively transported through the lipid bilayer of plant membranes. Some studies, however, indicate that the log Kow value of a chemical may not be the sole factor determining its tendency to be taken up and some compounds have been shown to be able to penetrate plant membranes despite a low log Kow (Renner, 2002). The capacity of a compound to be removed from water by a given plant, may also depend on other factors such as initial pollutant concentration, the anatomy and the root system of the plant (Chaudhry et al., 2002). In addition, very hydrophobic chemicals (log Kow > 3.5) are also candidates for phytostabilization and/or rhizosphere bioremediation by virtue of their long residence times in the root zone (USEPA, 2000; Dietz and Schnoor, 2001; Pilon-Smits, 2005).

Uptake has primary control over translocation, metabolism and phytotoxic action because the total amount of xenobiotic available for these processes is determined by the amount of compound absorbed by the plant. Metabolism influences both xenobiotic uptake and their phytotoxic action by either rendering the compound less or more active (Dietz and Schnoor, 2001; Kvesitadze et al., 2006).

4.2.1. What Happens to Organic Xenobiotics Once Taken up by the Plant?

Organic xenobiotics taken up by roots are translocated into different organs of the plants as a result of the physiological processes involved in the transport of nutrients. The main forces involved in this transport are related to the transpiration stream, i.e. transport of water and dissolved substances from roots to shoots, passing through vessels and tracheids located in the xylem (Kvesitadze et al., 2006).

The importance of the transpiration stream for the uptake and translocation of organics by plants is expressed in the following equation (Briggs et al., 1983; Dietz and Schnoor, 2001):

$$U = (TSCF)\ (T)\ (C) \tag{1}$$

where U is the rate of organic compound assimilation (mg day-1); T, the rate of plant transpiration, (L day-1); C, the organic compound concentration in the water phase (mg L-1); TSCF, the transpiration stream concentration factor, is a dimensionless ratio between the concentration of the organic compound in the liquid of the transpiration stream (xylem sap) and the bulk concentration in the root zone solution (Dietz and Schnoor, 2001; Doucette et al., 2005; Kvesitadze et al., 2006).

The TSCF has been extensively used in modeling of uptake and translocation of organic compounds in plants. With the possible exception of some hormone-like chemicals such as the phenoxy acid herbicides, there is no evidence of active uptake (TSCF > 1) of xenobiotic organic chemicals (Doucette et al., 2005). A chemical is said to be excluded (TSCF < 1) when its uptake is not directly proportional to water uptake (TSCF = 1), although the mechanism of uptake is still thought to be a passive process. However, factors such as membrane permeability and xylem sap solubility of the contaminant may limit the extent or kinetics of passive uptake (Doucette et al., 2005). Sorption and rapid metabolism of contaminants within the plant may also reduce xylem concentrations and keep measured TSCF values from reaching one (Doucette et al., 2005).

For organic chemicals, several empirical relationships between TSCF and the log Kow of the xenobiotic have been reported in which these values are related by characteristic bell-shaped gaussian curves (Briggs et al., 1983; Hsu et al., 1990; Sicbaldi et al., 1997; Burken and Schnoor, 1998; de Carvalho et al., 2007; Paraiba, 2007). These, again, suggest an optimal lipophilicity (corresponding to the maxima of the Gaussian curves) for uptake and translocation and infer that compounds which are either highly polar (log Kow < 0.5) or are highly lipophilic (log Kow > 3.5) will not be significantly taken up by plants. However, laboratory and field experiments with some xenobiotics such as 1,4-dioxane, MTBE, sulfolane and diisopropanolamine also suggest that these predictive schemes may not be applicable for some non-ionizable, highly water soluble organics (Aitchison et al., 2000; Rubin and Ramaswami, 2001; Groom et al., 2002; Chard et al., 2006).

4.2.2. Plant Detoxification Processes

Organic xenobiotics which penetrate the plant cells are exposed to plant's metabolic transformations that may lead to their partial or complete degradation or through which they may be transformed in less toxic compounds and bound in plant tissues (Korte et al., 2000; Kvesitadze et al., 2006).

Metabolism of foreign compounds in plant systems is generally considered to be a "detoxification" process that is similar to the metabolism of xenobiotic compounds in humans, hence the name "green liver" that is used to refer to these systems (Sandermann, 1994). Once an organic xenobiotic is taken up and translocated, it undergoes one or several phases of metabolic transformation, as is illustrated by the diagram in Figure 4.

Three possible phases of metabolic transformation of organic compounds in higher plants can be identified (Sandermann, 1994):

Phase I – Functionalization: involves a conversion/activation (oxidation, reduction or hydrolysis) of lipophilic xenobiotic compounds (Komives and Gullner, 2005; Eapen et al., 2007); in this phase the molecules of the hydrophobic compound acquire a hydrophilic functional group (e.g. hydroxyl, amine, carboxyl, sulphydryl) through enzymatic transformations. The polarity and water solubility of the compound increase as a result of these processes, which also causes an increased affinity to enzymes catalyzing further transformation (conjugation or deep oxidation (Korte et al., 2000; Kvesitadze et al., 2006)) by the addition or exposure of the appropriate functional groups. In the case of a low concentration, oxidative degradation of some xenobiotics to common metabolites of the cell and CO2 may take place. Following this pathway, a plant cell not only detoxifies the compound but also assimilates the resulting carbon atoms for cell needs. In case of a high concentration, full detoxification is not achieved and the contaminant is exposed to conjugation (Korte et al., 2000).

During this phase several different groups of enzymes are known to play an important role (Sandermann, 1992; Sandermann, 1994; Macek et al., 2000; Eapen et al., 2007). In plants, oxidative metabolism of the xenobiotics is mediated mainly by cytochrome P450 monooxygenase which is of crucial importance in the oxidative processes to bioactivate the xenobiotics into chemically reactive electrophilic compounds which subsequently form conjugates during Phase II. Peroxidases are another important group of enzymes, which help in the conversion of some of the xenobiotics. Peroxygenases may also be involved in the oxidation of some compounds. Nitroreductase is needed for the degradation of nitroaromatics and laccase for breaking up aromatic ring structures.

Phase I reactions are the first step needed to ultimately make a xenobiotic less toxic; those reactions modify the molecule to be ready for Phase II and Phase III reactions which further detoxify the chemical. However, if it already has a functional group suitable for Phase II metabolism, the compound can directly be used for Phase II without entering Phase I.

Phase II – Conjugation: involves conjugation of xenobiotic metabolites of Phase I (or the xenobiotics themselves when they already contain appropriate functional groups) to endogenous molecules (proteins, peptides, amino acids, organic acids, mono-, oligo- and polysaccharides, pectins, lignin, etc.) (Coleman et al., 1997; Korte et al., 2000; Dietz and Schnoor, 2001; Eapen et al., 2007); as result of conjugation, compounds of higher molecular weight are formed with greatly reduced biological activity and usually reduced mobility. The end products of Phase II are usually less toxic than the original molecules or Phase I derivatives.

Conjugation is catalyzed by transferases. Enzymes such as glutathione-S-transferases, glucosyl transferase and N-malonyl transferases are associated with Phase II (Eapen et al., 2007).

Conjugation of Phase I metabolites takes place in the cytosol, but it is harmful to accumulate these compounds in cytosol (Eapen et al., 2007).

Phase III – Compartmentalization: involves modified xenobiotics getting compartmentalized in vacuoles or getting bound to cell wall components such as lignin or hemicellulose (Coleman et al., 1997; Dietz and Schnoor, 2001; Eapen et al., 2007). In this phase (a potential final step in the non-oxidative utilization of xenobiotics) the conjugates are removed from vulnerable sites in cytosol and transported to sites where they may not interfere with cellular metabolism: soluble conjugates (with peptides, sugars, amino acids, etc.) are accumulated in vacuoles, whereas insoluble conjugates (coupled with pectin, lignin, xylan and other polysaccharide) are taken out of the cell and accumulated in plant cell walls (Sandermann, 1992; Sandermann, 1994; Eapen et al., 2007).

Phase III reactions are unique to plants because they do not excrete xenobiotics as animals do. Plants therefore, need to somehow remove the xenobiotic within their own system. ATP driven vacuolar transporters are the main enzymes involved in this phase and further processing of conjugates may take place in the vacuolar matrix (Eapen et al., 2007).

It is assumed that Phase III products are no longer toxic; however, this area of xenobiotic fate in plants is poorly understood, especially with reference to the identity of the sequestered products and any subsequent fate in herbivores who might consume those plants.

Metabolism of pesticides has already been extensively studied (Chaudhry et al., 2002; Coleman et al., 2002; Eapen et al., 2007). More recently, the metabolism of non-agricultural xenobiotics such as trichloroethylene (TCE), TNT, glyceroltrinitrate (GTN), PAHs, PCBs and other organic compounds has also been studied (Görge et al., 1994; Salt et al., 1998; Alkorta and Garbisu, 2001; Hannink et al., 2002; Eapen et al., 2007). It has been shown that most of these compounds are metabolized, but only a few chemicals appear to be fully mineralized. Studies applied to pharmaceutical substances, however, are very scarce until now (Huber et al., 2009) in spite of the great interest that such data represents for phytoremediation applications.

4.2.3. Phytotoxicity of Organic Xenobiotics

All plants have defense mechanisms to protect them from the negative effects of small quantities of foreign compounds. The relative rates of organic xenobiotics uptake, translocation, and metabolism usually determines whether or not these compounds will induce a plant response, which can be inferred from the plant's physiological, biochemical and molecular responses.

Physiological responses such as growth reduction, chlorosis and necrosis of tissues can usually be observed easily. Quantitative parameters can also be evaluated, which can provide an assessment of physiological toxic responses to xenobiotic stress, namely the plant's relative growth rate (RGR) or the photosynthetic pigments concentration in plant tissues. Alteration of these two parameters, have been observed for plants exposed to xenobiotics, sometimes compromising plant viability (Mishra et al., 2006).

The photosynthetic apparatus is one of the most important targets of stress in plants. Indeed, most of the metabolic responses induced by stress conditions have consequences on the aptitude of the plant to maintain an efficient light energy conversion (Rmiki et al., 1999). Alteration in the chlorophylls (total, a and b) and carotenoids contents have been reported in plants subjected to stress conditions (Ferrat et al., 2003). In general stressed plants tend to increase their carotenoid content to provide protection against the formation of free oxygen radicals. A decrease in total chlorophyll and in the ratio chlorophyll/carotenoids are often observed (Ferrat et al., 2003). These variations in photosynthetic pigments under exposure to trace metals and organic xenobiotics such as herbicides have been observed for various species (Ferrat et al., 2003).

Biochemical alterations are also induced by the presence of organic xenobiotics which lead to a production of reactive oxygen species (ROS). These chemical species are partially reduced forms of atmospheric oxygen (O_2). They typically result from the excitation of the triplet O_2 to form singlet oxygen (O_21) or from the transfer of one, two or three electrons to O_2 to form, respectively, superoxide radicals (•O_2-), hydrogen peroxide (H_2O_2) or O_23- (which dismutates into water and hydroxyl radicals, •OH) (Wojtaszek, 1997; Mittler, 2002; Apel and Hirt, 2004; Smirnoff, 2005). These are usually produced by plants as by-products of various metabolic pathways (such as photosynthesis and respiration) localized in different cellular compartments (predominantly in chloroplasts, mitochondria and peroxisomes) (Apel and Hirt, 2004).

Under physiological steady state conditions these molecules are scavenged by different antioxidative defense components that are often confined to particular compartments (Apel and Hirt, 2004). However, their overproduction can be triggered by external stress factors such as xenobiotics exposure. When exposed to xenobiotics, plants activate pathways to metabolize these foreign compounds which produce large amounts of ROS and may perturb the normal equilibrium between production and scavenging of ROS. As a result of these disturbances, intracellular levels of ROS may rapidly rise, thus posing a threat to the cell viability (Mittler, 2002; Masella et al., 2005).

The rapid and transient production of high quantities of ROS consequently results in what is called "oxidative burst" (Wojtaszek, 1997; Apel and Hirt, 2004). ROS, unlike the atmospheric oxygen, are capable of unrestricted oxidation of various cellular components and, if not controlled, have the ability to damage biomolecules (e.g. membrane lipid peroxidation, protein oxidation, enzyme inhibition, and DNA and RNA damage) and that can ultimately lead to the oxidative destruction of the cell (Mittler, 2002; Masella et al., 2005).

For these reasons, the ROS levels within the cells must be strictly controlled and kept within a narrow range. Plants cells have developed mechanisms to monitor and scavenge excessive amounts of ROS. Plants tolerance to pollutants is related to their capacity to cope with ROS over production.

Despite these problems, a steady-state of ROS is required within the cells because they also act as a signal for the activation of stress response and defense pathways. Thus, ROS can be viewed as cellular indicators of stress, and as secondary messengers involved in the stress-response signal transduction pathway. As such, the measurement of antioxidant enzymes activities has been used frequently for assessing environmental stress induced in plants by various pollutants (Mittler, 2002; Apel and Hirt, 2004).

Two different mechanisms are involved in ROS control: one that will enable the fine modulation of low levels of ROS for signaling purposes, and one that will enable the detoxification of excess ROS, especially during stress. Mechanisms of ROS detoxification exist in all plants and can be categorized as non-enzymatic (e.g. by flavanones, anthocyanins, carotenoids and ascorbic acid (AsA)) or as enzymatic. Major enzymatic ROS scavengers in plants include superoxide dismutase (SOD), ascorbate peroxidase (APX), glutathione peroxidase (GPX), and catalase (CAT) whose pathways are represented in Figure 5 (Mittler, 2002; Apel and Hirt, 2004; Geoffroy et al., 2004; Ashraf, 2009). The enzymes involved are present in different cell compartments and their expression is genetically controlled and regulated both by developmental and environmental stimuli, according to the needs for removing the ROS produced in the cells (De Gara et al., 2003).

SOD acts as the first line of defense against ROS, dismutating superoxide (O2-) to H2O2 (Figure 5a). APX, GPX, and CAT subsequently detoxify H2O2.

CAT, present in the peroxisomes of nearly all aerobic cells, can protect the cell from H2O2 by catalysing its decomposition into O2 and H2O (Mittler, 2002; Apel and Hirt, 2004) (Figure 5b). In contrast to CAT, APX requires an ascorbate and glutathione (GSH) regeneration system, the ascorbate-glutathione cycle (Figure 5d).

Detoxifiying H2O2 to H2O by APX occurs by oxidation of ascorbate to monodehydroascorbate (MDA) (Equation 1 in Figure 5d), which can be regenerated by MDA reductase (MDAR) using NAD(P)H as reducing agent (Equation 2 in Figure 5d). MDA can spontaneously dismutate into ascorbate and dehydroascorbate (DHA). Ascorbate regeneration is mediated by dehydroascorbate reductase (DHAR) driven by the oxidation of GSH to oxidized glutathione (GSSG) (Equation 3 in Figure 5d).

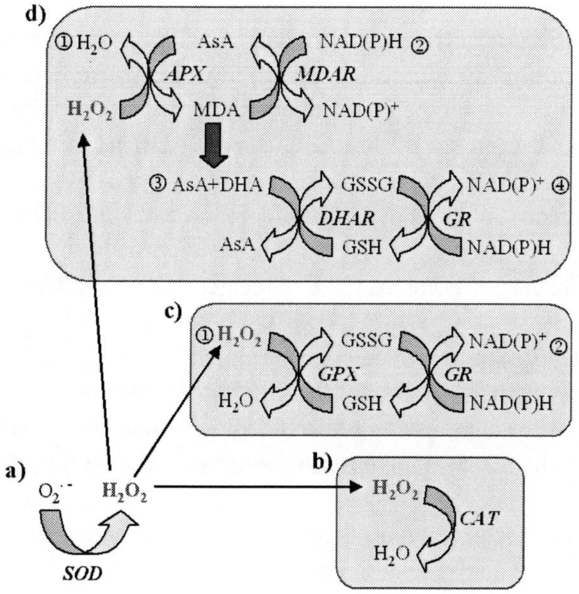

Figure 5. The main cellular pathways for ROS scavenging in plants. (a) Superoxide dismutase (SOD). (b) Catalase (CAT). (c) The glutathione peroxidase cycle. (d) The ascorbate-glutathione cycle. Abbreviations: AsA, ascorbate; APX, ascorbate peroxidase; MDA, monodehydroascorbate; MDAR, monodehydroascorbate reductase; DHA, dehydroascorbate; DHAR, dehydroascorbate reductase; GSH, glutathione; GSSG, oxidized glutathione; GPX, glutathione peroxidase; GR, glutathione reductase. (Adapted from Mittler (2002)).

Table 3. Detoxifying enzymes and respective ROS scavenging reactions (Wojtaszek, 1997; Mittler, 2002; Blokhina et al., 2003; Ashraf, 2009)

Enzyme	EC number	Location	Reaction catalyzed
Superoxide dismutase	1.15.1.1	Chol, Cyt, Mit, Per, Apo	O2 .- + O2 .- + 2H+ → 2 H2O2 + O2
Catalase	1.11.1.6	Per	2 H2O2 → O2 + 2H2O
Ascorbate peroxidase	1.11.1.11	Chol, Cyt, Mit, Per, Apo	2Asa + H2O2 → 2MDA + 2H2O (2MDA → AsA + DHA)
Guaiacol peroxidase	1.11.1.7	Cyt	Donor + H2O2 ↔ oxidized donor + 2H2O
Glutathione peroxidase	1.11.1.12	Cyt	2GSH + H2O2 ↔GSSG + 2H2O
Glutathione S-transferase	2.5.1.18	Cyt, Mit	RX+GSH ↔ HX + R-S-GSH*
MDA reductase	1.6.5.4	Chl, Mit, Per, Cyt	NADPH + MDA ↔ NAD(P)+ + AsA
DHA reductase	1.8.5.1	Chl, Mit, Per	2GSH + DHA ↔ GSSG + AsA
Glutathione reductase	1.6.4.2	Chl, Cyt, Mit	2NADPH + GSSG ↔ 2NADP+ + 2GSH

Abbreviations: Apo, apoplast; Chl, chloroplast; Cyt, cytosol; Mit, mitochondria; Per, peroxisome; * R may be an aliphatic, aromatic or herocyclic group; X may be a sulfate, nitrite or halite group.

Finally, glutathione reductase (GR) can regenerate GSH from GSSG using NAD(P)H as a reducing agent (Equation 4 in Figure 5d). Like APX, GPX also detoxifies H2O2 to H2O, but uses GSH directly as a reducing agent (Equation 1 in Figure 5c). The GPX cycle is closed by regeneration of GSH from GSSG by GR using NAD(P)H (Equation 2 in Figure 5c) (Wojtaszek, 1997; Mittler, 2002).

Unlike most organisms, plants have multiple genes encoding SOD and APX. Different isoforms are specifically targeted to chloroplasts, mitochondria, peroxisomes, as well as to the cytosol and apoplast (Table 3). Whereas GPX is located in cytosol, CAT is located mainly in peroxisomes (Table 3).

The extent of oxidative stress in a cell is determined by the concentrations of superoxide, hydrogen peroxide, and hydroxyl radicals. Therefore, the balance of SOD, APX, and CAT activities will be crucial for suppressing toxic ROS levels in a cell. Changing the balance of scavenging enzymes will induce compensatory mechanisms (Mittler, 2002; Apel and Hirt, 2004; Smirnoff, 2005).

In Table 3 a summary is presented of the several enzymes and reactions involved in the enzymatic ROS control and detoxification processes.

In the processes of detoxification and response against oxidative stress, phenolic compounds, which are ubiquitous plant secondary metabolites, may have an important role both in enzymatic as well as non-enzymatic mechanisms. Many phenolic compounds are used as substrates for antioxidant enzymes (and for the guaiacol peroxidase in particular) (Smirnoff, 2005). In addition, phenolic compounds have antioxidant properties on their own because their chemical structure enables them to quench radicals, which makes them also important players in the non-enzymatic control of the oxidative burst (Smirnoff, 2005).

The alteration of the levels of phenolic compounds is, therefore, a quantitative parameter which is complimentary to the evaluation of antioxidant enzymes activities to assess the oxidative stress induced by the plants exposure to xenobiotics.

The toxic effects caused in plants (including Typha spp.) by specific types of xenobiotic organic compounds (especially pesticides, but including other classes of compounds as well) have been extensively studied (Langan and Hoagland, 1996; Wilson et al., 2000; Amaya-Chavez et al., 2006; Olette et al., 2008). However, once again, oxidative stress induced by pharmaceuticals is still poorly studied and characterized, thus contributing to the general scarcity of data available for adequate design of phytoremediation solutions for pharmaceuticals contamination (Pomati et al., 2004; Boxall et al., 2006; Kong et al., 2007; Dordio ct al., 2009b).

CONCLUSION

Pollution caused by POPs is a matter of considerable concern as many of these substances have significant ecotoxicity and thus may negatively impact the environment and even present risks to human health. However, as awareness of the problem has arisen during the last decades, the realization that the conventional wastewater treatment processes were inefficient to deal with these types of pollutants and the need to also remediate sites that were already significantly contaminated has led to a search for new processes and technologies that could adequately reduce the presence or release of most of these substances to the environment. Some of the more efficient or traditionally used technologies that have been available have high costs which limit their application in most situations. As a low cost alternative, plants and associated rhizosphere microorganisms have over time been employed to treat wastewaters as well as remediate contaminated sites, in a variety of phytotechnologies where the targets to be cleaned up and the mechanisms in effect during the treatment may differ substantially.

Phytotechnologies have several advantages among which are the aesthetically pleasant installations and the usually good public acceptance, but the typically long periods required to achieve the remediation goals and the limitation to low concentrations of the pollutants due to the possible toxicity to the plants may in some cases deter its applicability. Despite some of its limitations, phytotechnologies have nevertheless been used with considerable success in the removal of varied types of POPs, both from contaminated soils and water. Several different types of mechanisms may be involved to different extents in the removal processes, some of which may be of the abiotic type but the most important ones being possibly of a biotic nature, due either from direct action of plants or from degradation by microorganisms stimulated by the plants.

Among the several types of phytotechnologies, constructed wetlands systems have been gaining an increasing popularity. The concerted action of plant species adapted to water saturated environments, microorganisms characteristic of these systems, and minerals of the support matrix, has shown good capabilities to deal with POPs through a variety of physical, chemical and biological processes. These systems are engineered in order to optimize these pollutant removal processes within a controlled environment. In order to achieve higher efficiencies, a good understanding of the mechanisms involved in the removal processes and the role played by each component are necessary so that components can be conveniently selected and design and operating conditions can be optimized. Some studies have already been conducted with this focus on understanding how CWS work and can be optimized. However, there is still a substantial amount of work that can and needs to be carried out in this area.

A subset of POPs which is part of a group of so-called emergent pollutants and has been raising special concern in the latest years is that of pharmaceutically active compounds. The need to treat this special class of compounds which were designed to provoke a biochemical effect and thus may cause particularly negative (and unpredicted) impacts has led to the study of CWS applications for the removal of this type of POP. This recent hot topic in wastewater treatment research shows the possibilities that are still open to the development of phytotechnologies, and applications of CWS in particular, for low cost solutions of emergent environmental problems. Studies conducted so far have shown the good perspectives that are presented for the use of these technologies. However, investigation of the mechanisms involved in the removal of these substances from the contaminated media, once again, may prove essential to attain the level of maturity of a wider application of these systems on a larger scale with reasonable results.

REFERENCES

Abhilash, P. C.; Jamil, S.; Singh, N. *Biotechnol. Adv.* 2009, 27, 474-488.

Aga, D. S. *Fate of Pharmaceuticals in the Environment and in Water Treatment Systems*; CRC Press: Boca Raton, FL, 2008.

Aitchison, E. W.; Kelley, S. L.; Alvarez, P. J. J.; Schnoor, *J. L. Water Environ. Res.* 2000, 72, 313-321.

Aken, B. V.; Correa, P. A.; Schnoor, *J. L. Environ. Sci. Technol.* 2009.

Alkorta, I.; Garbisu, C. *Bioresour. Technol.* 2001, 79, 273-276.

Amaya-Chavez, A.; Martinez-Tabche, L.; Lopez-Lopez, E.; Galar-Martinez, M. Chemosphere 2006, 63, 1124-1129.

Amon, J. P.; Agrawal, A.; Shelley, M. L.; Opperman, B. C.; Enright, M. P.; Clemmer, N. D.; Slusser, T.; Lach, J.; Sobolewski, T.; Gruner, W.; Entingh, *A. C. Ecol. Eng.* 2007, 30, 51-66.

Andreozzi, R.; Raffaele, M.; Nicklas, P. *Chemosphere* 2003, 50, 1319-1330.

Apel, K.; Hirt, H. *Annu. Rev. Plant Biol.* 2004, 55, 373-399.

Arnold, W. A.; McNeill, K. In *Analysis, fate and removal of pharmaceuticals in the water cycle*; Petrovic, M.; Barceló, D.; Eds.; Elsevier: Amsterdam, Netherlands, 2007; pp 361-385.

Ashraf, M. *Biotechnol. Adv.* 2009, 27, 84-93.

Ashton, D.; Hilton, M.; Thomas, K. V. *Sci. Total Environ.* 2004, 333, 167-184.

Bailey, H. C.; Elphick, J. R.; Krassoi, R.; Mulhall, A. M.; Lovell, A. J.; Slee, D. *J. Environ. Toxicol. Chem.* 2005, 24, 1773-1778.

Ballschmiter, K. Angew. *Chem. Int. Edit.* 1992, 31, 487-515.

Barceló, D.; Petrovic, M. *Emerging contaminants from industrial and municipal waste.* Ocurrence, Analysis and Effects; Springer-Verlag: Berlin, Germany, 2008.

Bendz, D.; Paxéus, N. A.; Ginn, T. R.; Loge, F. J. *J. Hazard. Mater.* 2005, 122, 195-204.

Benner, J.; Salhi, E.; Ternes, T.; von Gunten, U. *Water Res.* 2008, 42, 3003-3012.

Benotti, M. J.; Brownawell, B. J. *Environ. Sci. Technol.* 2007, 41, 5795-5802.

Benotti, M. J.; Trenholm, R. A.; Vanderford, B. J.; Holady, J. C.; Stanford, B. D.; Snyder, S. A. *Environ. Sci. Technol.* 2009, 43, 597-603.

Blankenberg, A. G.; Braskerud, B.; Haarstad, K. Int. J. *Environ. Anal. Chem.* 2006, 86, 225-231.

Blokhina, O.; Virolainen, E.; Fagerstedt, K. V. *Ann. Bot.* 2003, 91, 179-194.

Bolong, N.; Ismail, A. F.; Salim, M. R.; Matsuura, T. *Desalination* 2009, 239, 229-246.

Bouldin, J. L.; Farris, J. L.; Moore, M. T.; Smith, J.; Cooper, C. M. *Chemosphere* 2006, 65, 1049-1057.

Bourg, A. C.; Mouvet, C.; Lerner, D. N. Q. J. *Eng. Geol. Hydrogeol.* 1992, 25, 359-370.

Boxall, A. B. A.; Johnson, P.; Smith, E. J.; Sinclair, C. J.; Stutt, E.; Levy, L. S. *J. Agric. Food Chem.* 2006, 54, 2288-2297.

Braskerud, B. C.; Haarstad, K. *Water Sci. Technol.* 2003, 48, 267-274.

Briggs, G. G.; Bromilow, R. H.; Evans, A. A.; Williams, M. *Pestic. Sci.* 1983, 14, 492-500.

Brix, H. *Water Sci. Technol.* 1994, 29, 71-78.

Brix, H. *Water Sci. Technol.* 1997, 35, 11-17.

Burken, J. G.; Schnoor, J. L. *Environ. Sci. Technol.* 1998, 32, 3379-3385.

Carballa, M.; Omil, F.; Lema, J. M. *Chemosphere* 2008, 72, 1118-1123.

Chard, B. K.; Doucette, W. J.; Chard, J. K.; Bugbee, B.; Gorder, K. *Environ. Sci. Technol.* 2006, 40, 4788-4793.

Chaudhry, Q.; Schröder, P.; Werck-Reichhart, D.; Grajek, W.; Marecik, R. *Environ. Sci. Pollut. Res.* 2002, 9, 4-17.

Coleman, J. O. D.; BlakeKalff, M. M. A.; Davies, T. G. E. *Trends Plant Sci.* 1997, 2, 144-151.

Coleman, J.; Frova, C.; Schröder, P.; Tissut, M. *Environ. Sci. Pollut. Res.* 2002, 9, 18-28.

Collins, C.; Fryer, M.; Grosso, A. Environ. *Sci. Technol.* 2006, 40, 45-52.

Comeau, F.; Surette, C.; Brun, G. L.; Losier, R. *Sci. Total Environ.* 2008, 396, 132-146.

Conkle, J. L.; White, J. R.; Metcalfe, C. D. *Chemosphere* 2008, 73, 1741-1748.

Cooper, E. R.; Siewicki, T. C.; Phillips, K. *Sci. Total Environ.* 2008, 398, 26-33.

Cooper, P. F.; Job, G. D.; Green, M. B.; Shutes, R. B. E. Reed Beds and Constructed Wetlands for Wastewater Treatment; WRc Publications: Medmenham, Marlow, UK, 1996.

Corcoran, J.; Winter, M. J.; Tyler, *C. R. Crit. Rev. Toxicol.* 2010, 40, 287-304.

Crane, M.; Watts, C.; Boucard, *T. Sci. Total Environ.* 2006, 367, 23-41.

Cunningham, V. L.; Binks, S. P.; Olson, M. *J. Regul. Toxicol. Pharmacol.* 2009, 53, 39-45.

Dabrowski, J. M.; Bennett, E. R.; Bollen, A.; Schulz, R. *Chemosphere* 2006, 62, 204-212.

Daughton, C. G.; Ternes, T. A. *Environ. Health Perspect.* 1999, 107, 907-938.

Davies, L. C.; Pedro, I. S.; Ferreira, R. A.; Freire, F. G.; Novais, J. M.; Martins-Dias, S. *Water Sci. Technol.* 2008, 58, 2017-2023.

de Carvalho, R. F.; Bromilow, R. H.; Greenwood, R. *Pest Manag. Sci.* 2007, 63, 798-802.

De Gara, L.; de Pinto, M. C.; Tommasi, F. Plant Physiol. *Biochem.* 2003, 41, 863-870.

Dietz, A. C.; Schnoor, *J. L. Environ. Health Perspect.* 2001, 109, 163-168.

Doble, M.; Kumar, A. In *Biotreatment of Industrial Effluents*; Butterworth-Heinemann: Burlington, 2005; pp 241-253.

Dordio, A.; Pinto, J.; Dias, C. B.; Pinto, A. P.; Carvalho, A. J. P.; Teixeira, D. M. Int. *J. Environ. Anal. Chem.* 2009a, 89, 835-848.

Dordio, A.; Carvalho, A. J. P.; Teixeira, D. M.; Dias, C. B.; Pinto, A. P. *Bioresour. Technol.* 2010, 101, 886-892.

Dordio, A.; Carvalho, A. J. P.; Pinto, A. P.; Costa, C. T. In *Pesticide Research Trends;* Tennefy, A. B.; Ed.; Nova Science Publishers: Hauppauge, NY, USA, 2008.

Dordio, A. V.; Duarte, C.; Barreiros, M.; Carvalho, A. J. P.; Pinto, A. P.; da Costa, C. T. *Bioresour. Technol.* 2009b, 100, 1156-1161.

Dordio, A. V.; Teimão, J.; Ramalho, I.; Carvalho, A. J. P.; Candeias, A. *J. E. Sci. Total Environ.* 2007, 380, 237-246.

Dosnon-Olette, R.; Couderchet, M.; Eullaffroy, P. *Ecotox. Environ. Safe.* 2009, 72, 2096-2101.

Doucette, W. J.; Chard, J. K.; Moore, B. J.; Staudt, W. J.; Headley, J. V. *Microchem. J.* 2005, 81, 41-49.

Eapen, S.; Singh, S.; D'Souza, S. F. *Biotechnol. Adv.* 2007, 25, 442-451.

El Shahawi, M. S.; Hamza, A.; Bashammakh, A. S.; Al Saggaf, W. T. *Talanta* 2010, 80, 1587-1597.

Emblidge, J. P.; DeLorenzo, *M. E. Environ. Res.* 2006, 100, 216-226.

Enick, O. V.; Moore, M. M. *Environ. Impact Assess. Rev.* 2007, 27, 707-729.

Esplugas, S.; Bila, D. M.; Krause, L. G.; Dezotti, M. J. *Hazard. Mater.* 2007, 149, 631-642.

Etnier, E. L. *Regul. Toxicol. Pharmacol.* 1989, 9, 147-157.

Farré, M. l.; Pérez, S.; Kantiani, L.; Barceló, D. *Trac-Trends Anal. Chem.* 2008, 27, 991-1007.

Fent, K. In Pharmaceuticals *in the environment: sources, fate, effects and risks*; Kümmerer, K.; Ed.; Springer-Verlag: Berlin, Germany, 2008; pp 175-203.

Fent, K.; Weston, A. A.; Caminada, D. *Aquat. Toxicol.* 2006, 76, 122-159.

Ferrat, L.; Pergent-Martini, C.; Romeo, M. *Aquat. Toxicol.* 2003, 65, 187-204.

Fountoulakis, M. S.; Terzakis, S.; Kalogerakis, N.; Manios, T. Ecol. Eng. 2009, 35, 1702-1709.

Gan, S.; Lau, E. V.; Ng, H. K. *J. Hazard. Mater.* 2009, 172, 532-549.

Garrison, A. W.; Pope, J. D.; Allen, F. R. In *Identification and Analysis of Organic Pollutants in Water*; Keith, L. H.; Ed.; Ann Arbor Science Publishers: Ann Arbor, MI, USA, 1976; pp 517-556.

Gavrilescu, M. *Eng. Life Sci.* 2005, 5, 497-526.

Geoffroy, L.; Frankart, U.; Eullaffroy, P. *Environ. Pollut.* 2004, 131, 233-241.

Gerecke, A. C.; Scharer, M.; Singer, H. P.; Muller, S. R.; Schwarzenbach, R. P.; Sagesser, M.; Ochsenbein, U.; Popow, G. *Chemosphere* 2002, 48, 307-315.

Gessner, T. P.; Kadlec, R. H.; Reaves, R. P. *Ecol. Eng.* 2005, 25, 457-469.

Gomez, M. J.; Martinez Bueno, M. J.; Lacorte, S.; Fernandez-Alba, A. R.; Aguera, A. *Chemosphere* 2007, 66, 993-1002.

Görge, E.; Brandt, S.; Werner, D. *Environ. Sci. Pollut. Res.* 1994, 1, 229-233.

Groom, C. A.; Halasz, A.; Paquet, L.; Olivier, L.; Dubois, C.; Hawari, *J. Environ. Sci. Technol.* 2002, 36, 112-118.

Gross, B.; Montgomery-Brown, J.; Naumann, A.; Reinhard, M. *Environ. Toxicol. Chem.* 2004, 23, 2074-2083.

Grove, J. K.; Stein, O. R. *Water Res.* 2005, 39, 4040-4050.

Guil, M. D. H.; Petrovic, M.; Radjenovic, J.; Fernández-Alba, A. R.; Fernández-Alba, A. R.; Barceló, D. In *Analysis, fate and removal of pharmaceuticals in the water cycle*; Petrovic, M.; Barceló, D.; Eds.; Elsevier: Amsterdam, Netherlands, 2007; pp 451-474.

Haberl, R.; Grego, S.; Langergraber, G.; Kadlec, R. H.; Cicalini, A. R.; Martins-Dias, S.; Novais, J. M.; Aubert, S.; Gerth, A.; Thomas, H.; Hebner, A. *J. Soil Sediment.* 2003, 3, 109-124.

Halling-Sørensen, B.; Nors Nielsen, S.; Lanzky, P. F.; Ingerslev, F.; Holten Lützhøft, H. C.; Jørgensen, S. E. *Chemosphere* 1998, 36, 357-393.

Hannink, N. K.; Rosser, S. J.; Bruce, N. C. *Crit. Rev. Plant Sci.* 2002, 21, 511-538.

Hao, C. Y.; Lissemore, L.; Nguyen, B.; Kleywegt, S.; Yang, P.; Solomon, K. *Anal. Bioanal. Chem.* 2006, 384, 505-513.

Hao, C.; Clement, R.; Yang, P. *Anal. Bioanal. Chem.* 2007, 387, 1247-1257.

Haritash, A. K.; Kaushik, C. P. *J. Hazard. Mater.* 2009, 169, 1-15.

Heberer, T. Toxicol. *Lett.* 2002, 131, 5-17.

Henderson, K. L.; Belden, J. B.; Coats, J. R. *Environ. Sci. Technol.* 2007, 41, 4084-4089.

Hernando, M. D.; Heath, E.; Petrovic, M.; Barceló, D. *Anal. Bioanal. Chem.* 2006a, 385, 985-991.

Hernando, M. D.; Mezcua, M.; Fernández-Alba, A. R.; Barceló, D. *Talanta* 2006b, 69, 334-342.

Hignite, C.; Azarnoff, D. L. *Life Sci.* 1977, 20, 337-341.
Hsu, F. C.; Marxmiller, R. L.; Yang, A. Y. S. *Plant Physiol.* 1990, 93, 1573-1578.
Huber, C.; Bartha, B.; Harpaintner, R.; Schroder, P. Environ. *Sci. Pollut. Res.* 2009, 16, 206-213.
Hughes, J. B.; Shanks, J.; Vanderford, M.; Lauritzen, J.; Bhadra, R. *Environ. Sci. Technol.* 1996, 31, 266-271.
Hummel, D.; Loffler, D.; Fink, G.; Ternes, T. A. *Environ. Sci. Technol.* 2006, 40, 7321-7328.
Ikehata, K.; Naghashkar, N. J.; El Din, M. G. *Ozone-Sci. Eng.* 2006, 28, 353-414.
Imfeld, G.; Braeckevelt, M.; Kuschk, P.; Richnow, H. H. *Chemosphere* 2009, 74, 349-362.
ITRC. *Phytoremediation Decision Tree;* Interstate Technology and Regulatory Cooperation Work Group - Phytoremediation Work Team: Washington, DC, USA, 1999.
Jjemba, P. K. *Ecotox. Environ. Safe.* 2006, 63, 113-130.
Jones, K. C.; de Voogt, P. *Environ. Pollut.* 1999, 100, 209-221.
Jones, O. A. H.; Voulvoulis, N.; Lester, J. N. *Environ. Technol.* 2001, 22, 1383-1394.
Jones, O. A. H.; Voulvoulis, N.; Lester, J. N. *Crit. Rev. Environ. Sci. Technol.* 2005, 35, 401-427.
Joss, A.; Keller, E.; Alder, A. C.; Göbel, A.; McArdell, C. S.; Ternes, T.; Siegrist, H. *Water Res.* 2005, 39, 3139-3152.
Kadlec, R. H.; Wallace, S. D. *Treatment Wetlands*; CRC Press: Boca Raton, FL, USA, 2009.
Kasprzyk-Hordern, B.; Dinsdale, R. M.; Guwy, A. *J. Water Res.* 2008, 42, 3498-3518.
Kasprzyk-Hordern, B.; Dinsdale, R. M.; Guwy, A. *J. Water Res.* 2009, 43, 363-380.
Khetan, S. K.; Collins, T. *J. Chem. Rev.* 2007, 107, 2319-2364.
Kim, S. D.; Cho, J.; Kim, I. S.; Vanderford, B. J.; Snyder, S. A. *Water Res.* 2007, 41, 1013-1021.
Knight, R. L.; Kadlec, R. H.; Ohlendorf, H. M. *Environ. Sci. Technol.* 1999, 33, 973-980.
Komives, T.; Gullner, G. Z. *Naturforsch.* (C) 2005, 60, 179-185.
Kong, W. D.; Zhu, Y. G.; Liang, Y. C.; Zhang, J.; Smith, F. A.; Yang, A. *Environ. Pollut.* 2007, 147, 187-193.
Korte, F.; Kvesitadze, G.; Ugrekhelidze, D.; Gordeziani, M.; Khatisashvili, G.; Buadze, O.; Zaalishvili, G.; Coulston, F. *Ecotox. Environ. Safe.* 2000, 47, 1-26.
Kot-Wasik, A.; Debska, J.; Namiesnik, *J. Trac-Trends Anal. Chem.* 2007, 26, 557-568.
Koutsouba, V.; Heberer, T.; Fuhrmann, B.; Schmidt-Baumler, K.; Tsipi, D.; Hiskia, A. *Chemosphere* 2003, 51, 69-75.
Kümmerer, K. *Chemosphere* 2001, 45, 957-969.
Kümmerer, K. *Pharmaceuticals in the environment: sources, fate, effects and risks*; Springer-Verlag: Berlin, Germany, 2008.
Kümmerer, K. *J. Environ. Manage.* 2009, 90, 2354-2366.
Kuster, M.; López de Alda, M. J.; Hernando, M. D.; Petrovic, M.; Martín-Alonso, J.; Barceló, D. *J. Hydrol.* 2008, 358, 112-123.
Kvesitadze, G.; Khatisashvili, G.; Sadunishvili, T.; Ramsden, J. J. In *Biochemical Mechanisms of Detoxification in Higher Plants;* Kvesitadze, G.; Khatisashvili, G.; Sadunishvili, T.; Ramsden, J. J.; Eds.; Springer: Berlin, Germany, 2006; pp 103-165.
Langan, M. M.; Hoagland, K. D. *Bull. Environ. Contam. Toxicol.* 1996, 57, 307-314.
Larsen, T. A.; Lienert, J.; Joss, A.; Siegrist, H. J. *Biotechnol.* 2004, 113, 295-304.
Leclercq, M.; Mathieu, O.; Gomez, E.; Casellas, C.; Fenet, H.; Hillaire-Buys, D. *Arch. Environ. Contam. Toxicol.* 2009, 56, 408-415.

Lishman, L.; Smyth, S. A.; Sarafin, K.; Kleywegt, S.; Toito, J.; Peart, T.; Lee, B.; Servos, M.; Beland, M.; Seto, P. *Sci. Total Environ.* 2006, 367, 544-558.

Lofrano, G.; Nikolaou, A.; Kostopoulou, M.; Pagano, G.; Belgiorno, V.; Napoli, R. M. A. In *Xenobiotics in the Urban Water Cycle: Mass Flows, Environmental Processes, Mitigation and Treatment Strategies;* Fatta-Kassinos, D.; Bester, K.; Kümmerer, K.; Eds.; Springer: Dordrecht, Netherlands, 2010; pp 129-145.

Low, D.; Tan, K.; Anderson, T.; Cobb, G. P.; Liu, J.; Jackson, W. A. Ecol. Eng. 2008, 32, 72-80.

Macek, T.; Mackova, M.; Kas, *J. Biotechnol. Adv.* 2000, 18, 23-34.

Masella, R.; Di Benedetto, R.; Vari, R.; Filesi, C.; Giovannini, *C. J. Nutr. Biochem.* 2005, 16, 577-586.

Matamoros, V.; Arias, C.; Brix, H.; Bayona, *J. M. Environ. Sci. Technol.* 2007a, 41, 8171-8177.

Matamoros, V.; Garcia, J.; Bayona, *J. M. Environ. Sci. Technol.* 2005, 39, 5449-5454.

Matamoros, V.; Arias, C.; Brix, H.; Bayona, *J. M. Water Res.* 2009a, 43, 55-62.

Matamoros, V.; Bayona, *J. M. Environ. Sci. Technol.* 2006, 40, 5811-5816.

Matamoros, V.; Caselles-Osorio, A.; García, J.; Bayona, J. M. Sci. *Total Environ.* 2008a, 394, 171-176.

Matamoros, V.; García, J.; Bayona, J. M. *Water Res.* 2008b, 42, 653-660.

Matamoros, V.; Hijosa, M.; Bayona, J. M. *Chemosphere* 2009b, 75, 200-205.

Matamoros, V.; Puigagut, J.; García, J.; Bayona, J. M. *Chemosphere* 2007b, 69, 1374-1380.

Maurer, M.; Escher, B. I.; Richle, P.; Schaffner, C.; Alder, A. C. *Water Res.* 2007, 41, 1614-1622.

Miège, C.; Choubert, J. M.; Ribeiro, L.; Eusèbe, M.; Coquery, M. *Environ. Pollut.* 2009, 157, 1721-1726.

Mishra, S.; Srivastava, S.; Tripathi, R. D.; Kumar, R.; Seth, C. S.; Gupta, D. K. *Chemosphere* 2006, 65, 1027-1039.

Mittler, R. *Trends Plant Sci.* 2002, 7, 405-410.

Moore, M. T.; Bennett, E. R.; Cooper, C. M.; Smith, S.; Shields, F. D.; Milam, C. D.; Farris, J. L. *Agric. Ecosyst. Environ.* 2001, 87, 309-314.

Moore, M. T.; Cooper, C. M.; Smith, S.; Cullum, R. F.; Knight, S. S.; Locke, M. A.; Bennett, E. R. *Environ. Pollut.* 2009, 157, 250-256.

Moore, M. T.; Rodgers, J. H.; Cooper, C. M.; Smith, S. Environ. Pollut. 2000, 110, 393-399.

Moore, M. T.; Schulz, R.; Cooper, C. M.; Smith, S.; Rodgers, J. H. *Chemosphere* 2002, 46, 827-835.

Neumann, M.; Schulz, R.; Schafer, K.; Muller, W.; Mannheller, W.; Liess, M. *Water Res.* 2002, 36, 835-842.

Newman, L. A.; Reynolds, C. M. *Curr. Opin. Biotechnol.* 2004, 15, 225-230.

Nikolaou, A.; Meric, S.; Fatta, D. *Anal. Bioanal. Chem.* 2007, 387, 1225-1234.

Olette, R.; Couderchet, M.; Biagianti, S.; Eullaffroy, P. *Chemosphere* 2008, 70, 1414-1421.

Omari, K.; Revitt, M.; Shutes, B.; Garelick, H. *Water Sci. Technol.* 2003, 48, 275-281.

Osenbrük, K.; Gläser, H. R.; Knöller, K.; Weise, S. M.; Möder, M.; Wennrich, R.; Schirmer, M.; Reinstorf, F.; Busch, W.; Strauch, G. *Water Res.* 2007, 41, 3259-3270.

Palmer, P. M.; Wilson, L. R.; O'Keefe, P.; Sheridan, R.; King, T.; Chen, C. Y. *Sci. Total Environ.* 2008, 394, 90-102.

Paraiba, L. C. *Chemosphere* 2007, 66, 1468-1475.

Park, N.; Vanderford, B. J.; Snyder, S. A.; Sarp, S.; Kim, S. D.; Cho, *J. Ecol. Eng.* 2009, 35, 418-423.

Parrish, Z. D.; Banks, M. K.; Schwab, A. P. *Int. J. Phytoremediat.* 2004, 6, 119-137.

Perelo, L. W. *J. Hazard. Mater.* 2010, 177, 81-89.

Petrovic, M.; Barceló, D. *Analysis, fate and removal of pharmaceuticals in the water cycle*; Elsevier: Amsterdam, Netherlands, 2007.

Pilon-Smits, E. *Annu. Rev. Plant Biol.* 2005, 56, 15-39.

Pomati, F.; Netting, A. G.; Calamari, D.; Neilan, B. A. *Aquat. Toxicol.* 2004, 67, 387-396.

Putschew, A.; Jekel, M. In *Analysis, fate and removal of pharmaceuticals in the water cycle;* Petrovic, M.; Barceló, D.; Eds.; Elsevier: Amsterdam, Netherlands, 2007; pp 265-278.

Rabiet, M.; Togola, A.; Brissaud, F.; Seidel, J. L.; Budzinski, H.; Elbaz-Poulichet, *F. Environ. Sci. Technol.* 2006, 40, 5282-5288.

Radjenovic, J.; Petrovic, M.; Barceló, D. *Trac-Trends Anal. Chem.* 2007, 26, 1132-1144.

Ralf, S.; Matt, T. M.; Erin, R. B.; Jerry, L. F.; Sammie, S., Jr.; Charles, M. C. *Environ. Toxicol. Chem.* 2003, 22, 1262-1268.

Reddy, K. R.; DeLaune, R. D. *Biogeochemistry of wetlands: science and applications*; CRC Press: Boca Raton, FL, USA, 2008.

Reichenberger, S.; Bach, M.; Skitschak, A.; Frede, H. G. *Sci. Total Environ.* 2007.

Renner, *R. Environ. Sci. Technol.* 2002, 36, 410A-413A.

Richardson, M. L.; Bowron, J. M. J. Pharm. *Pharmacol.* 1985, 37, 1-12.

Rmiki, N.-E.; Lemoine, Y.; Schoefs, B. In *Handbook of plant and crop stress*; Pessarakli, M.; Ed.; CRC Press, 1999; pp 465-482.

Robinson, I.; Junqua, G.; Van Coillie, R.; Thomas, O. Anal. Bioanal. *Chem.* 2007, 387, 1143-1151.

Rogers, I. H.; Birtwell, I. K.; Kruzynski, G. M. *Water Poll. Res. J. Can.* 1986, 21, 187-204.

Rose, M. T.; Sanchez-Bayo, F.; Crossan, A. N.; Kennedy, I. R. *Chemosphere* 2006, 63, 1849-1858.

Rubin, E.; Ramaswami, A. *Water Res.* 2001, 35, 1348-1353.

Salt, D. E.; Smith, R. D.; Raskin, I. Annu. Rev. Plant Physiol. *Plant Mol. Biol.* 1998, 49, 643-668.

Sandermann, H. *Trends Biochem. Sci.* 1992, 17, 82-84.

Sandermann, H. *Pharmacogenet.* 1994, 4, 225-241.

Sanderson, H.; Johnson, D. J.; Reitsma, T.; Brain, R. A.; Wilson, C. J.; Solomon, K. R. Regul. *Toxicol. Pharmacol.* 2004, 39, 158-183.

Scholz, M.; Lee, B. h. *Int. J. Environ. Stud.* 2005, 62, 421-447.

Schroder, P.; Collins, C. *Int. J. Phytoremediat.* 2002, 4, 247-265.

Schulz, R. *J. Environ. Qual.* 2004, 33, 419-448.

Schulz, R.; Peall, S. *K. C. Environ. Sci. Technol.* 2001, 35, 422-426.

Sicbaldi, F.; Sacchi, G. A.; Trevisan, M.; Delre, A. A. M. *Pestic. Sci.* 1997, 50, 111-119.

Singer, A. C.; Crowley, D. E.; Thompson, I. P. *Trends Biotechnol.* 2003, 21, 123-130.

Singh, O. V.; Jain, R. K. *Appl. Microbiol. Biotechnol.* 2003, 63, 128-135.

Smirnoff, N. *Antioxidants and reactive oxygen species in plants*; Blackwell Publishing Ltd: Oxford, UK, 2005.

Snyder, S. A.; Adham, S.; Redding, A. M.; Cannon, F. S.; DeCarolis, J.; Oppenheimer, J.; Wert, E. C.; Yoon, Y. Desalination 2007, 202, 156-181.

Stackelberg, P. E.; Furlong, E. T.; Meyer, M. T.; Zaugg, S. D.; Henderson, A. K.; Reissman, D. B. *Sci. Total Environ.* 2004, 329, 99-113.

Stottmeister, U.; Wiessner, A.; Kuschk, P.; Kappelmeyer, U.; Kastner, M.; Bederski, O.; Muller, R. A.; Moormann, *H. Biotechnol. Adv.* 2003, 22, 93-117.

Stumpf, M.; Ternes, T. A.; Wilken, R. D.; Silvana, V. R.; Baumann, *W. Sci. Total Environ.* 1999, 225, 135-141.

Sun, T. R.; Cang, L.; Wang, Q. Y.; Zhou, D. M.; Cheng, J. M.; Xu, *H. J. Hazard. Mater.* 2010, 176, 919-925.

Sundaravadivel, M.; Vigneswaran, S. *Crit. Rev. Environ. Sci. Technol.* 2001, 31, 351-409.

Susarla, S.; Medina, V. F.; McCutcheon, *S. C. Ecol. Eng.* 2002, 18, 647-658.

Tang, X.; Eke, P. E.; Scholz, M.; Huang, S. *Bioresour. Technol.* 2009, 100, 227-234.

Tauxe-Wuersch, A.; De Alencastro, L. F.; Grandjean, D.; Tarradellas, *J. Water Res.* 2005, 39, 1761-1772.

Ternes, T. A. *Water Res.* 1998, 32, 3245-3260.

Ternes, T. A.; Bonerz, M.; Herrmann, N.; Teiser, B.; Andersen, H. R. *Chemosphere* 2007, 66, 894-904.

USEPA. *Introduction to phytoremediation*; EPA/600/R-99/107; Office of Research and Development: Cincinnati, OH, USA, 2000.

USEPA. *Phytoremediation field studies database for chlorinated solvents, pesticides, explosives, and metals;* Office of Superfund Remediation and Technology Innovation: Washington, DC, USA, 2004.

USEPA; USDA-NRCS. *A Handbook of Constructed Wetlands*. Volume 1: General Considerations; USEPA Region III with USDA-NRCS: Washington, DC, USA, 1995.

Van Aken, B. *Curr. Opin. Biotechnol.* 2009, 20, 231-236.

Vanderford, M.; Shanks, J. V.; Hughes, *J. B. Biotechnol. Lett.* 1997, 19, 277-280.

Vangronsveld, J.; Herzig, R.; Weyens, N.; Boulet, J.; Adriaensen, K.; Ruttens, A.; Thewys, T.; Vassilev, A.; Meers, E.; Nehnevajova, E.; van der, L. D.; Mench, M. Environ Sci. *Pollut. Res. Int.* 2009, 16, 765-794.

Velagaleti, *R. Drug Inf. J.* 1997, 31, 715-722.

Vieno, N.; Tuhkanen, T.; Kronberg, *L. Water Res.* 2007, 41, 1001-1012.

Vymazal, *J. Ecol. Eng.* 2009, 35, 1-17.

Vymazal, J.; Brix, H.; Cooper, P. F.; Green, M. B.; Haberl, R. *Constructed wetlands for wastewater treatment in Europe*; Backhuys Publishers: Leiden, The Netherlands, 1998.

Waggott, A. In *Chemistry in water reuse*; Cooper, W. J.; Ed.; Ann Arbor Science Publishers: Ann Arbor, MI, USA, 1981; pp 55-99.

Watts, C. D.; Crathorne, M.; Fielding, M.; Steel, C. P. In *Analysis of organic micropollutants in water*; Angeletti, G.; Bjørseth, A.; Eds.; D. Reidel Pub. Co.: Dordrecht, Netherlands, 1983; pp 120-131.

Weigel, S.; Kallenborn, R.; Hühnerfuss, *H. J. Chromatogr.* A 2004, 1023, 183-195.

Weishaar, J. A.; Tsao, D.; Burken, J. G. *Int. J. Phytoremediat.* 2009, 11, 509-523.

Williams, *J. B. Crit. Rev. Plant Sci.* 2002, 21, 607-635.

Wilson, P. C.; Whitwell, T.; Klaine, *S. J. Arch. Environ. Contam. Toxicol.* 2000, 39, 282-288.

Wojtaszek, P. *Biochem.* J. 1997, 322, 681-692.

Xia, H.; Ma, X. *Bioresour. Technol.* 2006, 97, 1050-1054.

Zhang, Y.; Geißen, S. U.; Gal, C. *Chemosphere* 2008, 73, 1151-1161.

Zhang, Z. L.; Zhou, *J. L. J. Chromatogr.* A 2007, 1154, 205-213.

Zodrow, *J. J. Remediat.* J. 1999, 9, 29-36.
Zorita, S.; Mårtensson, L.; Mathiasson, *L. Sci. Total Environ.* 2009, 407, 2760-2770.
Zounkova, R.; Odraska, P.; Dolezalova, L.; Hilscherova, K.; Marsalek, B.; Blaha, *L. Environ. Toxicol. Chem.* 2007, 26, 2208-2214.
Zuccato, E.; Castiglioni, S.; Fanelli, *R. J. Hazard. Mater.* 2005, 122, 205-209.

In: Xenobiotics: New Research
Editors: Saul F. Castaneda and Mauro L. Emerson
ISBN: 978-1-61942-616-0

Chapter 7

THE USE OF BACTERIAL BIOSENSORS TO DETERMINE THE TOXICTY OF NANOMATERIALS AND OTHER XENOBIOTICS

R. I. Dams**, A. Biswas, A. Olesiejuk, M. Gómez, M. M. Murcia, N. Christofi and T. Fernandes
Pollution Research Unit, Edinburgh Napier University,
Merchiston Campus, Edinburgh EH10 5DT, Scotland, UK

ABSTRACT

It is widely accepted that the current and planned increase in commercial development of nanotechnology will lead to pronounced releases of nanomaterials (NM) in the environment. In this study we aim to evaluate the toxicity of silver nanoparticles and some chlorinated phenol compounds by using a common sludge bacterium, Pseudomonas putida (originally isolated from activated sludge) as biosensor in bioluminescence assays. The results of the toxicity testing were expressed as IC50 values which represents the amount of toxicants required to reduce light output by 50% and calculated using a statistical program that was developed in-house. The bacterium carrying a stable chromosomal copy of the lux operon (luxCDABE) was able to detect toxicity of ionic and particulate silver over short term incubations ranging from 30-240 min. The IC50 values obtained at different time intervals showed that highest toxicity (lowest IC50) was obtained after 90 min incubation for all toxicants and this is considered the optimum incubation for testing. The data show that ionic silver is most toxic followed by nanosilver particles with microsilver particles being least toxic. Release of nanomaterials is likely to have an effect on the activated sludge process as indicated by this study using a common sludge bacterium involved in biodegradation of organic wastes. Among the chlorinated phenol compounds, 3,5 dichlorophenol showed the highest toxicity and phenol being the least toxic. Among the hydroxylated compounds tested, benzoquinone showed to be the most toxic compound. Understanding the fate and transport of phenolic compounds and transformation products in removal treatment plants is relevant in evaluating the impact of discharge in the environment and in developing a

* Author for correspondence. E-mail address: rosemedero@yahoo.co.uk Phone/fax: +44 0131-455-2291.

program for pollution control. Our results demonstrate that the use of a bacterial biosensor as P. putida BS566::luxCDABE, native from a highly polluted environment, provides a robust, early warning system of acute toxicity which could lead to process failure. This strain is suitable for toxicity monitoring in a highly polluted industrial waste water treatment streams and it has the potential to inform on upstream process changes prior to their impacting upon the biological remediation section.

Keywords: Bacterial biosensors, Pseudomonas putida, silver nanoparticles, wastewater treatment, phenol compounds, ecotoxicity

1. Introduction

Bacterial Biosensors

Bioluminescence is associated with the emission of light by living microorganisms and it plays a very important role in real time process monitoring. Biosensors are able to monitor very low levels of chemicals, can work in complex matrices and have very fast response times. Furthermore, it requires short times of analysis and provide low cost of assays, portable equipment, real-time measurements. When the reporter lux gene is fused to a promoter regulated by the concentration of a compound of interest, this concentration can be quantitatively analyzed by detecting the bioluminescence intensity. On the other hand, when the reporter is fused to promoters that are continuously expressed as long as the organism is alive and metabolically active, it will be proper for evaluating the total toxicity of contaminant.

Recombinant bioluminescent biosensing cells have been widely used to determine the toxicity of several xenobiotics as herbicide paraquat (Belkin et al., 1997), phenolic compounds (Ben-Israel et al., 1998; Gu and Choi, 2001; Boyd et al., 2001) and its degradation byproducts (Choi and Gu, 2003) and recently to test the toxicity of oxide nanoparticles to bacteria and crustaceans (Heinlaan et a., 2008) to protozoa (Mortimer et al., 2003), to microalgae (Aruoja et al., 2009), to protozoa and crustaceans in natural waters (Blinova et al., 2010).

Nanoparticles Toxicity

The knowledge of the ecotoxicology of nanoparticles (NP) to bacteria and other microbes is still limited, even though some manufactured nanoparticles (NP; materials with three dimensions between 1-100nm; Bridges et al., 2007) such as silver and titanium, which are constantly released into the environment, are known as antibacterial agents. As such it is essential that technology that fully assesses their effects on natural microbial entities, and on biogeochemical cycling in the environment, is available. Clearly there is a concern that these novel materials could be released into the environment, and that there may be releases from products that are in current use. However, we are only just starting to explore their ecotoxicology and environmental chemistry.

The increased commercial development of nanotechnology has the potential release of such nanoparticles in the environment, however, knowledge on their fate and effects on biota in natural habitats is still lacking, particularly using real systems such aquatic and marine waters and terrestrial systems. A particular knowledge gap relates to the effect of NP on the ubiquitous microbial community of the planet that is responsible for the recycling of organic material and the continued fertility of aquatic and terrestrial systems. Bacteria perform many critical roles required for normal ecosystem function and productivity, such as carbon and nitrogen cycling. Toxicity of nanoparticles to bacteria has caused many concerns. Interactions between bacteria and NPs may provide us with more information about the impact of NPs once released into the ecosystem. At the same time, bacteria as single cell organisms are good test models to study the NPs' toxicity and to know how the NPs affect the cell/organism function.

Although is not clear which mechanism is responsible for the toxic effect of nanoparticles on bacterial cells, quite a lot of information is available for nano-sized particles due to their use as bactericides. Sondi and Salopek-Sondi (2004) observed aggregates of silver nanoparticles in dead cells of E. coli using scanning electron microscopy. Other studies have observed the citotoxicity of iron-based nanoparticles toward Escherichia coli where the authors (Auffan et al., (2008) found out that nanoparticles containing zerovalent iron were toxic to the bacteria probably due to the generation of reactive oxygen species.

Sinha et al., (in press) studied the effect of silver and zinc nanoparticles towards mesophilic and halophilic bacteria cells. They observed that nanotoxicity was more pronounced on halophilic Gram negative bacteria than mesophilic bacteria cells. Also, it was observed by the authors (Sinha et al., 2010) that Gram positive halophilic bacteria showed a resistance towards both silver and zinc nanoparticles.

Among the oxide nanoparticles tested (aluminium, silicon, titanium and zinc) Jiang et al., (2009) found out that zinc was the most toxic to Bacillus subtilis, E. coli and Pseudomonas fluorescens. Clearly, toxicity is also species dependent and it can be associated with characteristics of certain bacterial species. For instance, Kim et al., (2007) observed a severe inhibitory effect on the growth of yeast and E.coli and a mild effect on Staphylococcus aureus. Siejak and Frackowiak (2007) have showed that the intensity of fluorescence of Cianobacterium synechocytis strongly diminished in the presence of 30nm silver nanoparticles.

One of the consequences of the increased utilization of nanomaterials is the release of these materials to the environment and consequently the amounts of nanowaste should increase. Source of nanomaterials maybe from the collection systems in municipalities where huge amounts of nanoparticles are release daily. The amount of nanoparticles reaching soil and natural waters depends on the fraction of wastewater that is effectively treated. A simplified pathway has been described by Bystrzejewska-Piotrowska et al., (2009) from nanotechnology to nanowaste, where unbound nanoparticles may be released from disposed or residue paints, cosmetics or pharmaceuticals, other nanoproducts, textiles or coatings may form composites. Toxic ions (from metallic nanoparticlers such as silver) may be released due to leaching.

Silver nanoparticles is well known for its antibacterial activity and have become one of the nanomaterials most used in consumer product (Maynard and Michelson, 2006), it is considered as the most prevalent of engineered materials (Rejeski and Lekas, 2008) and is likely that nanowaste should increase and therefore enter the wastewater treatment plants.

Blaser et al. (2008) pointed out that silver released to wastewater is incorporated into sewage sludge and may spread further on agricultural fields where will mainly stay in the top layer of soils (Hou et al. 2005). Land filling of sewage sludge may allow silver to leach into subsoil and groundwater. Estimation of silver load in sewage sludge and its microorganisms growth inhibition has been predicted. Blaser et al., (2008) predicted that an expected silver concentration in sewage treatment plant range from 2 μg L-1 to 18 μg L-1. Shafer et al., (1998) reported a range of ~ 2 to 4 μg L-1 of silver in sewage treatment plants treating common wastewater and a much higher load from industrial discharges (from 24 to 105 μg L-1). Choi et al., (2008) have demonstrated that Ag-NP have an inhibitory effect on the growth of autotrophic and heterotrophic bacteria in wastewater treatment plants. In these studies, Choi et al., (2008) found out that silver ion was the most toxic species (among silver nanoparticles, silver ions and silver loride colloids) to inhibit heterotrophic growth. Therefore, its release into the environment as waste has arisen serious concern. Certainly, nanomaterials do not behave in the same way as normal waste ans therefore there is a need for a more suitable and fast system which allows a early warning about the entrance of such nanomaterials into the waste water treatment. The current standard wastewater treatment technologies might not be suitable for removing NMs from the effluents, thus providing an escape route for dissolved chemicals as it has been postulated from Leppard et al., 2003. Recently, Westerhoff et al., (2008) demonstrated the wastewater treatment systems' inability to remove NMs from drinking water, therefore implying the potential presence of NMs in drinking water with an exposure pathway to humans.

The bioluminescence bioassay here performed is able to offer this possibility where in manner of minutes or few hours is possible to monitor the presence of these nanoparticles, specially silver nanoparticles, the object of this study.

Phenol Compounds

Chlorophenols are ranked as severe environmental pollutants and are important intermediates in the chemical industry (Fallmann et al., 1999) and have been used as biocides or as starting components for pesticide production (McAllister et al.,1996; Litchfield and Rao,1998; Chi and Huang, 2002). Highly chlorinated phenols have been listed as priority pollutant by the US Environmental Protection Agency (Keith and Telliard,1979). Chloro-substituted phenols and cresols are known to be toxic to humans as well as to aquatic life (Keith and Telliard, 1979). They often occur in industrial wastewaters and solid waste leachates causing their recalcitrance to biological treatments. Chlorinated compounds can be removed from the environment by physicochemical processes, biological degradation including various aerobic, anaerobic, and combined aerobic–anaerobic biological processes. And during their transformation, many byproducts are produced by partial degradation, which may result in increasing toxicity levels (Paton et al., 1997). Trichlorophenol and dichlorophenol have been found as intermediate compounds during dechlorination of PCP in horizontal-flow anaerobic immobilized biomass reactors (Damianovic et al. 2009) and PCP anaerobic degradation pathway (Madsen and Aamand, 1990). The production of intermediates from a partial dechlorination of PCP can generate even more toxic compounds as 3,4,5-trichlorophenol (TCP), which was found to be more toxic than PCP (Wu et al.,

1989). The chemical 2,4,6-TCP has been considered one of the most toxic chlorophenols (Eker and Kargi, 2007).

Hydroxylated compounds such as catechol, hydroquinone, resorcinol and benzoquinone may be produced in the oxidative transformation of phenols (Fukushima et al., 2002; Gorska et al. 2009) and 4-chlorocathecol has been identified as intermediate in a *meta* cleavage of 4-chlorophenol (Hollender et al., 1997). Also, under ozonation treatment of PCP, benzoquinone and hydroquinone were identified as intermediate compounds (Hong and Zeng, 2002). Thus, removal of the original compounds can be considered as only a partial measure of the efficiency of the treatment.

It is generally accepted that in the assessment of toxicity of environmental pollutants, a range of bioassays are required to examine the variability in a toxic response involving organisms of different trophic levels. The same specifically applies to microorganisms and, bacteria in particular, where different species can respond differently to toxic chemicals. Whole microbial cell biosensors are now widely used as research tools in the testing of substances likely to elicit cytotoxic and genotoxic events, and, in the determination of bioavailability of chemicals (Belkin, 2007). There are many advantages using biosensors as monitoring very low levels of chemicals, working with complex matrices and have very fast response times (Dennison and Turner,1995). They embrace genetically engineered bacteria that have a toxicant detecting gene that is coupled with a reporter gene (e.g. luminescence gene such as lux or luc) capable of producing a detectable response on activation.

Table 1. Stock Solutions' Concentrations of Chlorinated Phenol and Intermediate Compounds

Compound	Stock solution (concentration g L^{-1})
Phenol	5 g/l
4-chlorophenol	1g/l
3,5 dichlorophenol	1g/l
2,4,6 trichlorophenol	1g/l
PCP	1g/l
4-chlorocatechol	1g/l
3,5 dichlorophenol	1g/l
Cathecol	0.500 g/l
Chlorocathecol	0.500 g/l
Benzoquinone	0.500 g/l
Chlorohidroquinone	0.500 g/l
Hydroquinone	0.500 g/l
Resorcinol	0.500 g/l
Chlororesorcinol	0.500 g/l
1,2,4 THB	0.500 g/l

In this ecotoxicity study we have focused on highly chlorinated phenols as pentachlorophenol, 2,4,6 trichlorophenol, 3,5 dichlorophenol and monosubstituted 4-chlorophenol and phenol due to their environmental relevance as pollutants. Phenolic compounds exert a toxic effect on microorganisms by disrupting energy transduction either by uncoupling oxidative phosphorylation or by inhibiting electron transport (Escher et al., 1996). Substituted phenols act by destroying the electrochemical proton gradient by transporting protons back across the membrane and/or inhibiting electron by binding to specific components of the electron transport chain (Escher et al., 1996).

As the luminescence of lux-marked bacterial biosensors depends on the products of the electron transport chain for light production, inhibition of this process due to chlorophenol toxicity will result in a decrease in light output.

In this study we performed ecotoxicological testing using a genetically-modified Pseudomonas isolated from a polluted, phenolic-rich, wastewater treatment system by transposon mutagenesis (Wiles et al., 2003). The Pseudomonas carries a stable chromosomal copy of the lux operon (luxCDABE) derived from Photorhabdus luminescens with continuous output of light.

Several compounds have been tested: chlorinated phenol compounds and some common by-products of degradation of phenolic compounds as hydroquinone, cathecol, chlorohydroquinone and benzoquinone. Silver materials in the ionic form, nanoparticles (35nm) and microparticles (0.6-1.6 microns).

2. Material and Methods

2.1. Chemicals

All of the chemicals used were analytical grade.

Phenol Compounds

Sodium Salt Pentachlorophenol (PCP) and Phenol were purchased from Sigma Chemical Company (USA); 3,5 dichlorophenol, 2,4,6 Trichlorophenol, and 4 Chlorophenol were purchased from Aldrich, Madison, Wis. 4-chlorocatechol (97%), resorcinol (99%), 4-chlororesorcinol (98%), chlorohydroquinone (85%) and p-benzoquinone (98%) were obtained from Aldrich. 1,2,4 trihydroxibenzene (THB), hydroquinone (99%), catechol (99%) were purchased from Sigma.

Stock solutions of PCP, 3,5 dichlrophenol, 4-chlorophenol, phenol, catechol, 4-chlorocatechol, resorcinol, 4-chlororesorcinol, hydroquinone, chlorohydroquinone, p-benzoquinone, 1,2,4 THB were freshly prepared in 0.85% saline solution. Stock solutions of 2,4,6 trichlorophenol was prepared in 0.2N NaOH solution. Working solutions were double diluted externally and then added to 96 well black microtitre plates used for the bioluminescence bioassays. Table I shows the stock solutions' concentrations used in the ecotoxicity tests.

Silver Species

Silver powder nanoparticles (average size: 35nm, 99.5% metal basis, spherical morphology and cubic crystallographic structure) and microparticles (average size: 0.6-1.6 microns) were obtained from Nanoamor (Nanostructured and Amorphous Materials Inc, Texas, USA).

Stock solutions of silver ion ($AgNO_3$), silver nanoparticles (Ag-NP) and silver microparticles (Ag-MP) were freshly made in 20 ml Universal flasks and placed into an ultrasonic bath (XB6 Grant Instruments Cambridge Ltd, UK) at 25 kHz, 250C for 30 minutes. Two fold dilutions were externally prepared of these solutions and added to the 96 well black microtitre plates (Sterling, Caerphilly, UK). Silver ion working solutions concentrations ranged from 0.23 μg L-1 to 2500 μg L-1. Silver nanoparticles solutions concentrations ranged from 0.195 mg L-1 to 200 mg L-1 and silver microparticles solutions concentrations ranged from 1.46 mg L-1 to 1500 mg L-1. Two different stabilisers were added to the nanoparticles and microparticles working solutions: 0.1% citric acid, 0.1% BSA (bovine serum albumin) and for comparison solutions with no stabiliser also were used. Previous studies have used BSA for stabilisation of ZnO nanoparticles (Brayner et al., 2006) and also as a carbon black nanomaterial stabiliser in suspension (Foucaud et al., 2007). Thus improving stability of particle suspension by decreasing the extent of particle agglomeration and settling over time (Foucaud et al., 2007). Citric acid is known to act as a chelating agent and may thus be able to also act to quench toxicity of dissolved metal toxicants and it has been found to reduce agglomeration of particles (Chu et al., 2002) thus improving particle distribution and response. All working solutions were light protected and used within 30 minutes of preparation. In order to verify no shading effects of the particles on the bacterial cells, light output was measured before and after addition of particles. No shading effects were determined.

2.2. Media and Growth Conditions

Organism

The bacterial strain used in this study, P. putida BS566::luxCDABE was constructed based upon chromosomal expression of the luxCDABE operon derived from an entomopathogenic nematode symbiont, Photorhabdus luminescens (Winson et al., 1998). Originally isolated from the treatment system (Whiteley et al., 2001), this reporter organism encompassing a dynamic xenobiotic sensing range, suitable for placement around an industrial processing system to monitor remediation in multiple compartments.. Cultures were grown in Luria-Bertani (LB) broth, containing 100 mgL-1 Kanamycin, overnight at 26oC with shaking (200rpm) to late exponential stage. Prior to the assay, cultures were diluted to approximately 107 cells/ml and regrown under the same conditions for two to three generations without Kanmycin. When OD (optical density) reached 0.2 (approximately 10 8 cell/ml) toxicity tests were carried out.

2.3. Biosensor Assay

Luminescence measurements were undertaken using a 96-well plate luminometer (FLUOstar Optima 1 and 2, BMG Labtech, UK) in 96 well black microtitre plates (Sterling, Caerphilly, UK) whereby each well contained bacterial inoculum and toxicant at the required concentration in 100 μL volumes, using an integration time of 1 s at a temperature of 28°C. Reading was taken at every 30 for 240 min. Control wells containing LB broth with P. putida

BS566::luxCDABE were run and changes in toxicity for the test systems are expressed as percentages of the control. Luminescence values were expressed in the instrument's arbitrary relative light units (RLU). The maximal response ratios were the highest ratios of luminescence in the sample-containing wells to luminescence in wells containing untreated cells determined during a specified period: 30, 90, 180 and 240 min (Belkin et., 1996).

Inhibitory concentration which represents 50% inhibition of light output (IC50) related to control was assessed for all toxicants tested. All experiments were run at least 3 times (most of 4 times) at different dates with different batches.

2.4. Calculation of IC_{50} (IC- Inhibitory Concentration) Values

The IC values are calculated using a statistical program that was developed in-house. The program fits a three parameter logistic model to the logarithm of the concentration by weighted least squares. The parameters are the initial response, the slope and the intercept. It is assumed that the response would decline to zero at sufficiently high concentrations. The initial response effectively uses the information from both the controls (if present) and low concentrations. The weights used are taken to be proportional to the fitted response but with adjustments for high and low responses; this is to protect against bias due to "hormesis" effects (stimulatory effects causing increased light output when challenged with low toxicant concentrations) and the effective omission of data respectively.

2.5. Data Analysis

For error analysis, all of the experiments were conducted three times on different plates. Data from at least eight wells were used for one concentration and coefficients of variation (CV) between independent assays were calculated using Microsoft Excell 97. Differences among treatments were tested using a two-way analysis of variance (ANOVA) to determine which treatments were statistically different ($P < 0.05$).

3. Results and Discussion

Phenol Compounds

Luminescence responses of the engineered strain P. putida BS566::luxCDABE was assessed using different concentrations of chlorinated phenol compounds of environmentally relevance and some intermediate compounds from their transformation. Luminescence activity was calculated as residual activity when compared to uninhibited samples, and expressed as a percentage of this control. This reporter was found to demonstrate a proportional decay in luminescence after incubation of 4h. Inhibitory concentration (IC_{50}) for each compound tested resulting in luminescence decay to 50% of the control luminescence was assessed.

Using the biosensor P. putida BS566::luxCDABE, IC_{50} values were determined (Table 2) for PCP, 2,4,6 trichlorophenol, 3,5 dicholorophenol, 4 chlorophenol, phenol, and the intermediate compounds: cathecol, chlorocathecol, benzoquinone, chlorohidroquinone, hydroquinone, chlororesorcinol, resorcinol and 1,2,4 THB.

Calculated coefficients of variation (CV) between independent assays were found to be between 2% and 16% (data not shown), which were lower than reported for another toxicity assays using Pseudomonas spp.(7 – 18%) (Brown et al. 1996; Paton et al. 1995), demonstrating the reproducibility and reliability of the developed toxicity assay.

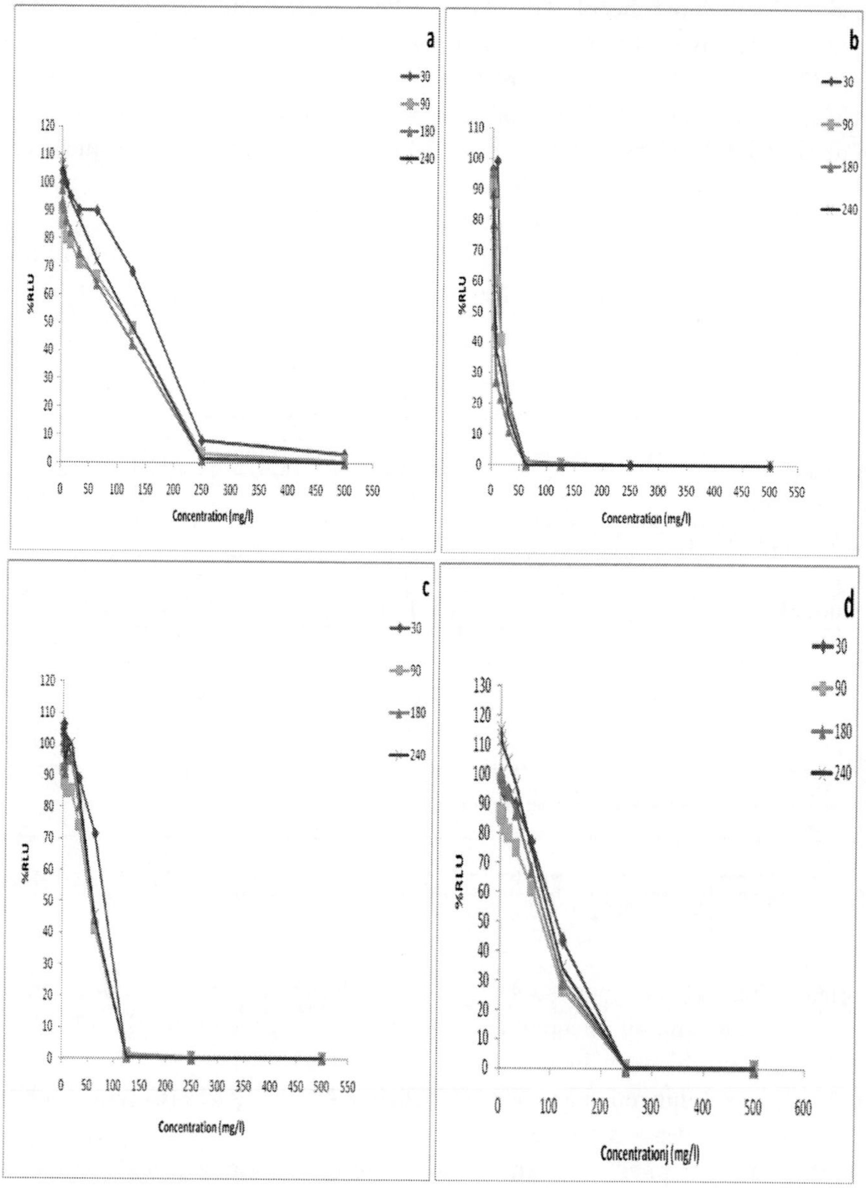

Figure 1. Light output reduction by P. putida BS566::luxCDABE when challenged with 4-Chlorophenol (a), 3,5 Dichlorophenol (b), mg L-1 2,4,6 Trichlorophenol (c) and PCP (d) after 30, 90, 80 and 240 min. Mean of three replicates with different batches. Coefficient of variation 12% among independent assays.

Figure 1 shows the light output reduction by P. putida BS566::luxCDABE when challenged with phenol compounds: 4- Chlorophenol; 3,5 Dichlorophenol; 2,4,6 Trichlorophenol and PCP. Overall, the predicted toxicity of all phenolic compounds indicated that 3,5 dichlorophenol was statistically the most toxic compound (<0.5). The order of toxicity to P. putida was: 3,5 dichlorophenol > 2,4,6 trichlorophenol> PCP> 4 chlorophenol. Figure 2 shows the luminescence reduction by P. putida when challenged with phenol. This organism showed a high tolerance to phenol. The IC50 value for phenol after 30 min of exposure to this toxicant was 437 mg L-1 (Table 2), which is about 87 fold greater than those determined for 3,5 dichlorophenol. After 4 h of exposure the IC50 found for growth inhibition of P. putida was 225 mg L-1, which was close to the value of 244 mg L-1 in a 6h test found by Slabbert (1986) in a 6h test using P. putida.

The IC_{50} values (Table 2) found for 2,4,6 trichlorophenol toxicity was 6.3 fold greater than that determined for phenol (P<0.05) after 30 min of exposure. After 90 min it dropped to ~3,5 and so remained until the end of the test (4h).

Table 2. IC_{50} ($mg\ l^{-1}$) Values for Light Emission Reduction by P. Putida BS566:: LUXCDABE after 30, 90, 180 and 240 Min

	IC_{50} values ($mg\ l^{-1}$)			
Time (min)	30	90	180	240
Phenol	437	237	218	225
4-chlorophenol	141	133	124	123
3,5 dicholorophenol	5	2,5	2,5	2,5
2,4,6 trichlorophenol	69	64	62	62
PCP	106	90	78	74
Chlorocathecol	160	115	93	66
Hydroquinone	159	393	325	300
Resorcinol	941	350	266	245
Cathecol	397	245	275	270
Benzoquinone	0.9	1.10	1.60	1.30
chlorohidroquinone	102	171	189	200
Chlororesorcinol	227	142	157	176
1,2,4 THB	41	79	88	122

Values presented are an average of at least 3 independent experiments carried out with different batches. Standard deviation between 2 and 16 %.

Chlorinated phenol compounds as tri and di chlorophenol are common intermediates among removal treatments of phenolic compounds such as pentachlorophenol. For instance, the pentachlorophenol biodegradation pathway by Burkholderia cepacia AC1100 (Zeng and Wackett, 2008) and Sphingomonas chorophenolicum ATCC 39723 (Copley, 2000) showed that through oxidative cleavage of the original compound, hidroquinones, trichlorophenol and dichlorophenol are generated as intermediates. Our results showed that within a 30 min bioluminescent assay is possible to determine the high toxicity of the intermediate compounds when comparing with the original compound. Also, showed that monochlorophenol was less toxic than di, trichlorophenol and pentrachlorophenol. Other species of *Pseudomonas fluorescens* and *Burkholderia Rasc* c2 (Boyd et al., 2001) used as biosensors also showed a greater sensibility to dichlorophenols and trichlorophenols than those determined for monochlorophenols. Chlorine substitution adds electrophilicity, resulting in reactive toxicity. Additionally, increasing chlorination increases the dissociation constant, making phenol derivatives more acidic (Paulus, 1993) and more polar due the presence of a strong hydrogen bonding group (-OH) (Cronin and Schultz, 1998).

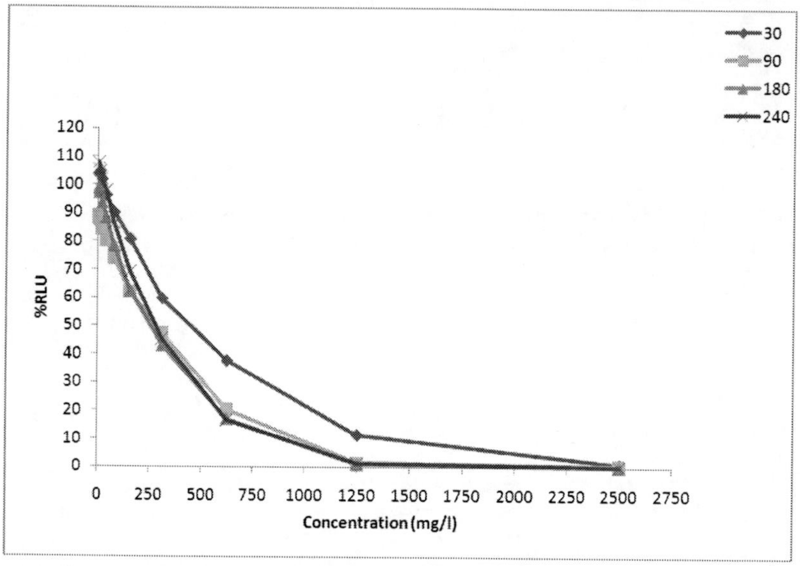

Figure 2. Light output reduction by P. putida BS566: luxCDABE when challenged with phenol after 30, 90, 80 and 240 min. Mean of three replicates with different batches. Coefficient of variation 7% among independent assays.

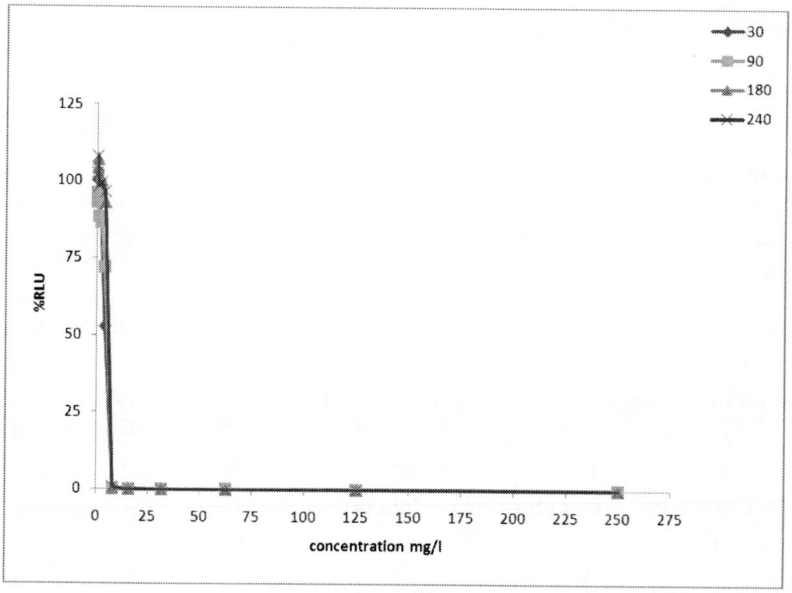

Figure 3. P. putida BS566:luxCDABE light output reduction when challenged with 500 mg L-1 Benzoquinone after 30, 90, 80 and 240 min. Mean of three replicates with different batches. Coefficient of variation 8 % among independent assays.

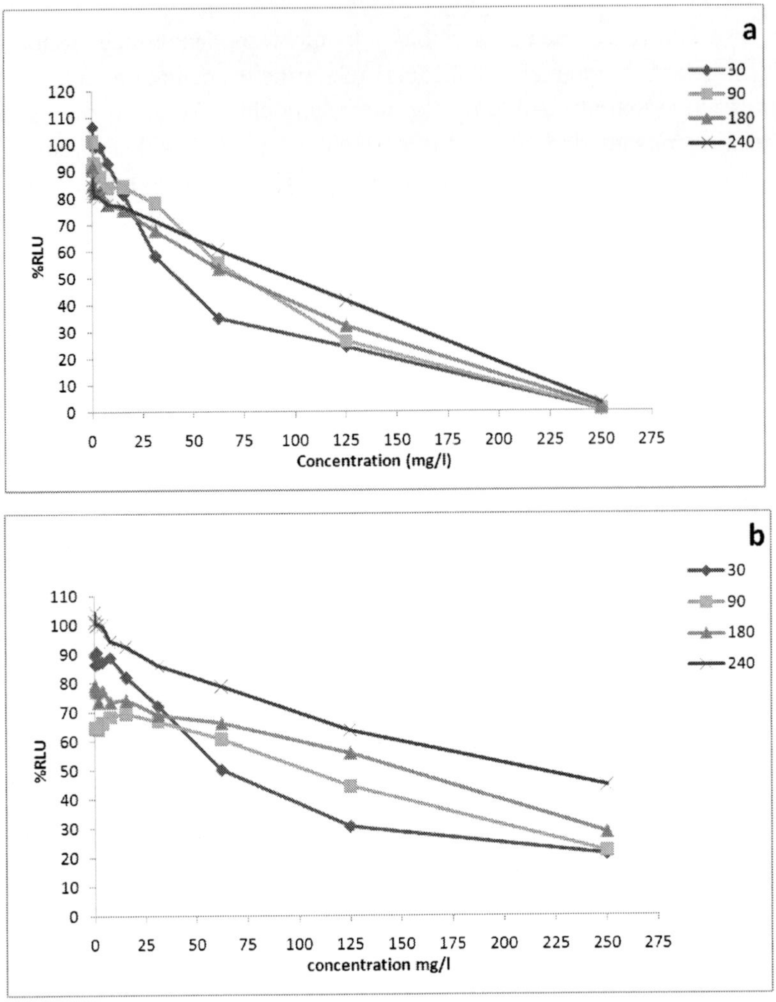

Figure 4. Light output reduction by P. putida BS566::luxCDABE when challenged with THB (a) and chlorohidroquinone after 30, 90, 80 and 240 min. Mean of three replicates with fifferent batches. Coefficient of variation 11% among independent assays.PCP and 4-chlorophenol toxicity was about 4 and 3 folder greater than that determined for phenol ($P<0.05$) after 30 min of exposure (Table 2) after 30 min of exposure, respectively.

In this study, byproducts originated from 4-chlorophenol photodegradation studies formerly carried out in our laboratories (Gomez et al., 2010) such as phenol, cathecol,benzoquinone, resorcinol, hydroquinone and others were tested for its toxicity. Fenton's reaction generates hydroxyl-radicals (OH) by means of the reaction of H_2O_2 with ferrous ion, which produces a range of intermediates upon treatment of aromatic and chloroaromatic compounds, including chlorophenols. The elementary reaction produces cyclohexadienyl radicals, which upon stabilization yield the corresponding quinones (Bunce et al., 1997; Chen and Pignatello, 1997; Kang et al., 2002; Pera-Titus et al., 2004). Figure 3 shows the light reduction by *P.* putida BS566::luxCDABE when challenged with benzoquinone. In this study, among the byproductos tested, benzoquinone is far the most toxic compound. The order of toxicity is: benzoquinone> 1,2,4 THB> chlorohidroquinone> hydroquinone> chlorocathecol> chlororesorcinol> cathecol> resorcinol (Table 2).

Figures 4-6 show the light reduction by P. putida BS566::luxCDABE when challenged with THB, chlorohydroquinone, hydroquinone, chlorocathecol, chlororesorcinol, cathecol and resorcinol. Most of the byproducts showed no residual toxicity after 4 h of exposure (THB, chlorohidroquinone, hydroquinone, chlororesorcinol, cathecol and resorcinol. However, benzoquinone and chlorocathecol after 4 h of exposure showed a residual toxicity in the order of 94 and 2 fold greater (Table 2), respectively, when comparing with the original compound 4-chlorophenol. Hydroxylated and carbonyl compounds are typically involved in the contaminant degradation, and low molecular weight organic acids are usually detected as a residual of the oxidation (Mills and Hoffmann, 1993; Stefan and Bolton, 1998). Kim et al., (2007) suggested that the observed PCP post-treatment toxicity might be due to toxic PCP byproducts, which may include polychlorinated dibenzodioxins/furans,tetrachloro-*p*-benzoquinone, and other intermediates. Tetrachlorohydroquinone, tetrachlorobenzoquinone and tetrachlorocatechol have been reported previously as PCP intermediates of TiO2 photo-oxidation, UV photodegradation and ozonation (Benitez et al., 2003; Hong and Zeng, 2002; Hirvonen et al., 2000; Luo et al., 2008; Weavers et al., 2000). It has been reported that complete mineralization into carbon dioxide and inorganic is obtained only with prolonged treatment, even though the half-life of the original contaminant may be very short (Sundstrom et al., 1989; Mills and Hoffmann, 1993). In that context, removal of the original compounds is only a partial measure of the efficiency of the treatment. The degradation products formed in the oxidation processes are mainly low molecular weight oxygenated and less toxic, more biodegradable than the original compounds (Miller *et al.* 1988) as observed for most of the intermediate compounds in this study (Table II). Previous studies in our laboratories (Gomez et., 2010) showed that when 4-chlorophenol was treated with excimer lamp only (without hydrogen peroxide), toxic concentrations of several byproducts, including hydroquinone, benzoquinone, resorcinol, chlorohydroquinone, remained in the medium after treatment, while hydrogen peroxide improved the removal of photoproducts. The residual oxidation products can persist after treatment because of their low reactivity towards the oxidants (Arnold et al., 1995). Consequently, the potential formation of persistent or toxic intermediates should be evaluated if the partial oxidation fulfilled the criteria for discharge to the subsequent stage of the treatment process or into the environment.

Thus, understanding the fate and transport of phenolic compounds and transformation products in removal treatment plants is relevant in evaluating the impact of discharge in the environment and in developing a program for pollution control.

Silver Materials

IC_{50} values following challenge with $AgNO_3$, Ag-NP and Ag-MP are shown in Table 3. Calculated coefficients of variation (CV) between independent assays were found to be between 1% and 15%. It is well known that silver ion and silver based compounds are highly toxic to microorganisms and showing strong biocide effects to many bacteria species (Zhao and Stevens, 1998; Sondi and Salopek-Sondi, 2004; Brayner et al., 2006; Pal et al., 2007; Choi et al., 2008; Jiang et al., 2009).

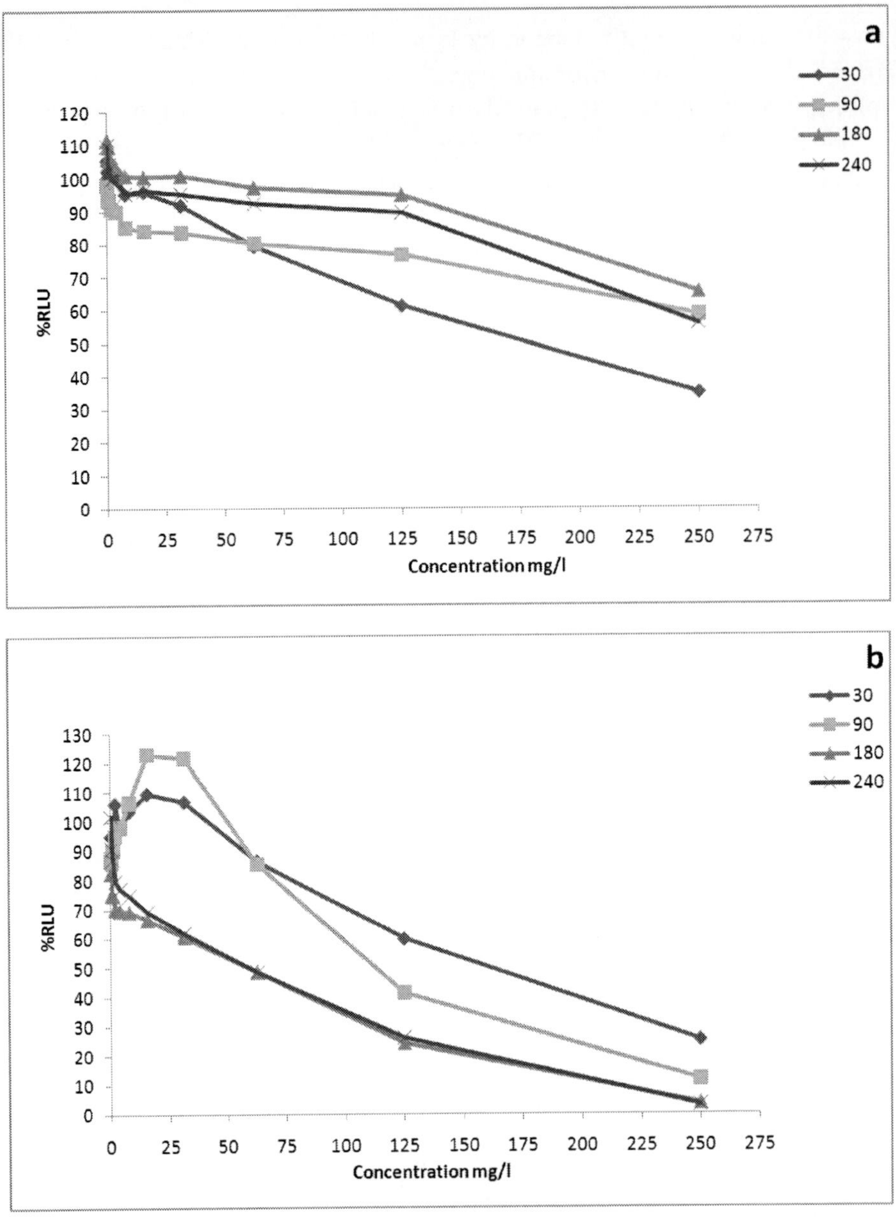

Figure 5. Light output reduction by P. putida BS566: luxCDABE when challenged with Hidroquinone (a) and chlorocathecol (b) after 30, 90, 80 and 240 min. Mean of three replicates with fifferent batches. Coefficient of variation 8 % among independent assays.

Figure 7 shows the light output reduction by P. putida BS566::luxCDABE when challenged with 2500μg L-1 Silver ion. Among the silver species tested, AgNO3 is by far the most toxic to P. putida in this study highlighting the action of ionic Ag+ ($P<0.05$).

Figures 8-9 show the light output reduction by P. putida BS566::luxCDABE when challenged with Ag nanoparticles and Ag microparticles. When using BSA as stabilizer, Ag nanoparticles showed to be statistically more toxic than Ag microparticles ($P<0.05$). The same was observed when using citric acid as stabilizer.

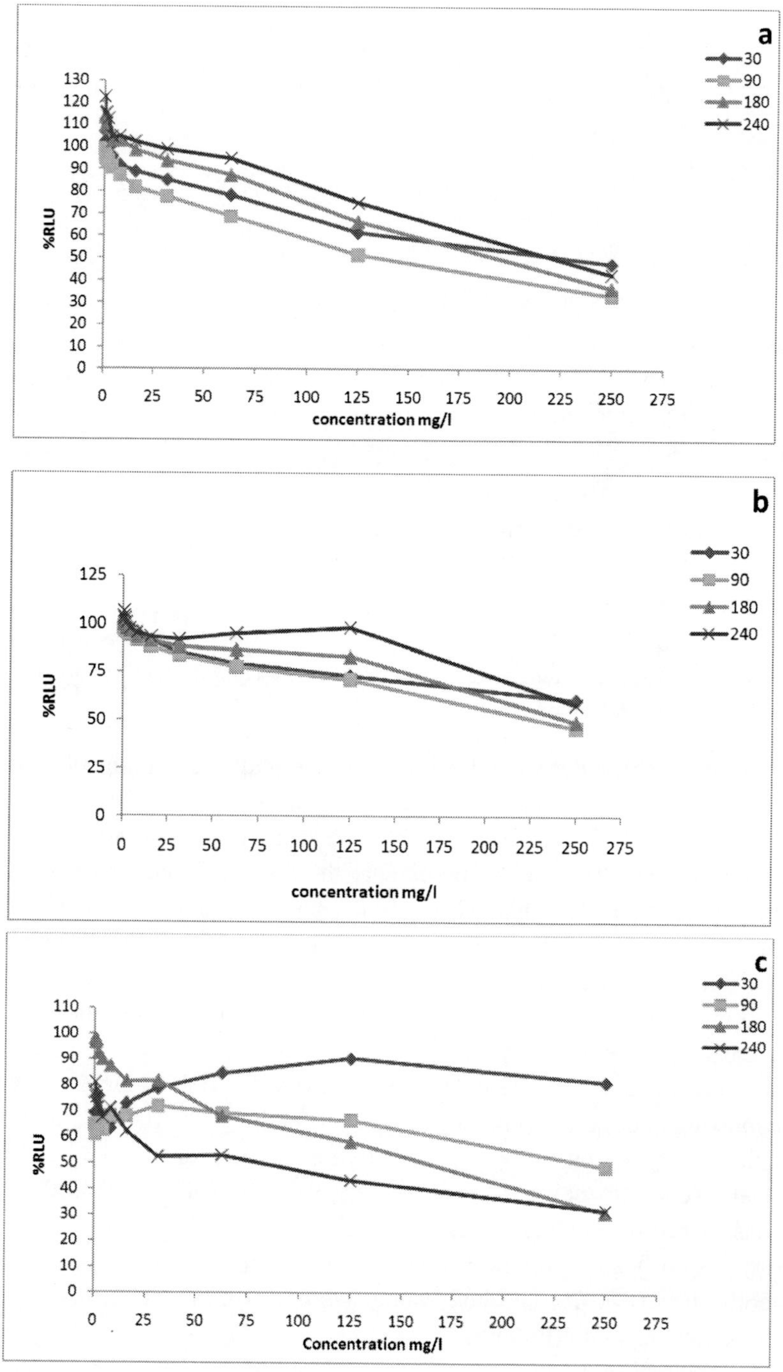

Figure 6. Light output reduction by P. putida BS566::luxCDABE when challenged with Chlororesorcinol (a), cathecol (b) and resorcinol (c) after 30, 90, 80 and 240 min. Mean of three replicates with fifferent batches. Coefficient of variation 8 % among independent assays.

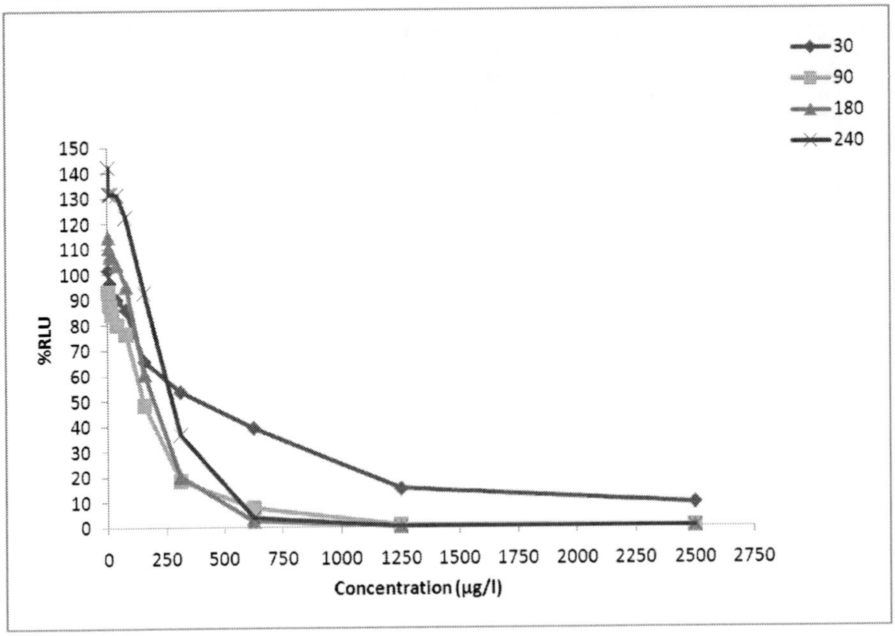

Figure 7. Light output reduction by P. putida BS566::luxCDABE when challenged with 2500µg L^{-1} Silver ion after 30, 90, 80 and 240 min. Mean of three replicates with different batches. Coefficient of variation 15% among independent assays.

Highest toxicity (Table 3) was obtained with the assay after 90 min incubation and indeed this was the case for all silver species tested with or without stabilisation. The order in toxicity was Ag+>Ag-NP (35 nm)>Ag-MP (0.6-1.6 µm). If we consider the 90 min assay results, that show the highest toxicity, to compare the data, it is seen that Ag-NP are nearly 200 times less toxic that Ag+, with Ag-MP ~3000 times less toxic in non-stabilised systems ($P<0.05$). The effect with Ag-NP was more pronounced in BSA systems with a calculated IC50 value ~4 times statistically lower than Ag-NP with citric acid ($P<0.05$). Both stabilisers appear to perform, increasing toxicity perhaps through better dispersion of the NP providing more surface area for Ag to have an effect. This however may not be the case as citric acid may be just as effective in preventing agglomeration. Citric acid is an effective chelating/complexing agent for metals in solution and perhaps its effect on the toxicity value is due to this fact acting to immobilise Ag+ released in solution or those on surfaces. The use of different stabilisers and their effect on toxicity values must be assessed particularly if laboratory bioassay results will have significance in wastewater discharge consents.

There was no significant difference in the IC50 value obtained for Ag-MP with BSA and citric acid stabilisation ($P>0.05$) and both values were ~2 times statistically lower than Ag-MP tested without stabilisation ($P<0.05$).

The antimicrobial effect is related to the amount and the rate of silver released by NP. Is has been proposed that ionised silver binds to cell membrane proteins and severe structural changes occur in the bacterial cell wall leading to cell distortion and death (Lansdown et al., 2002; Castellano et al., 2007).

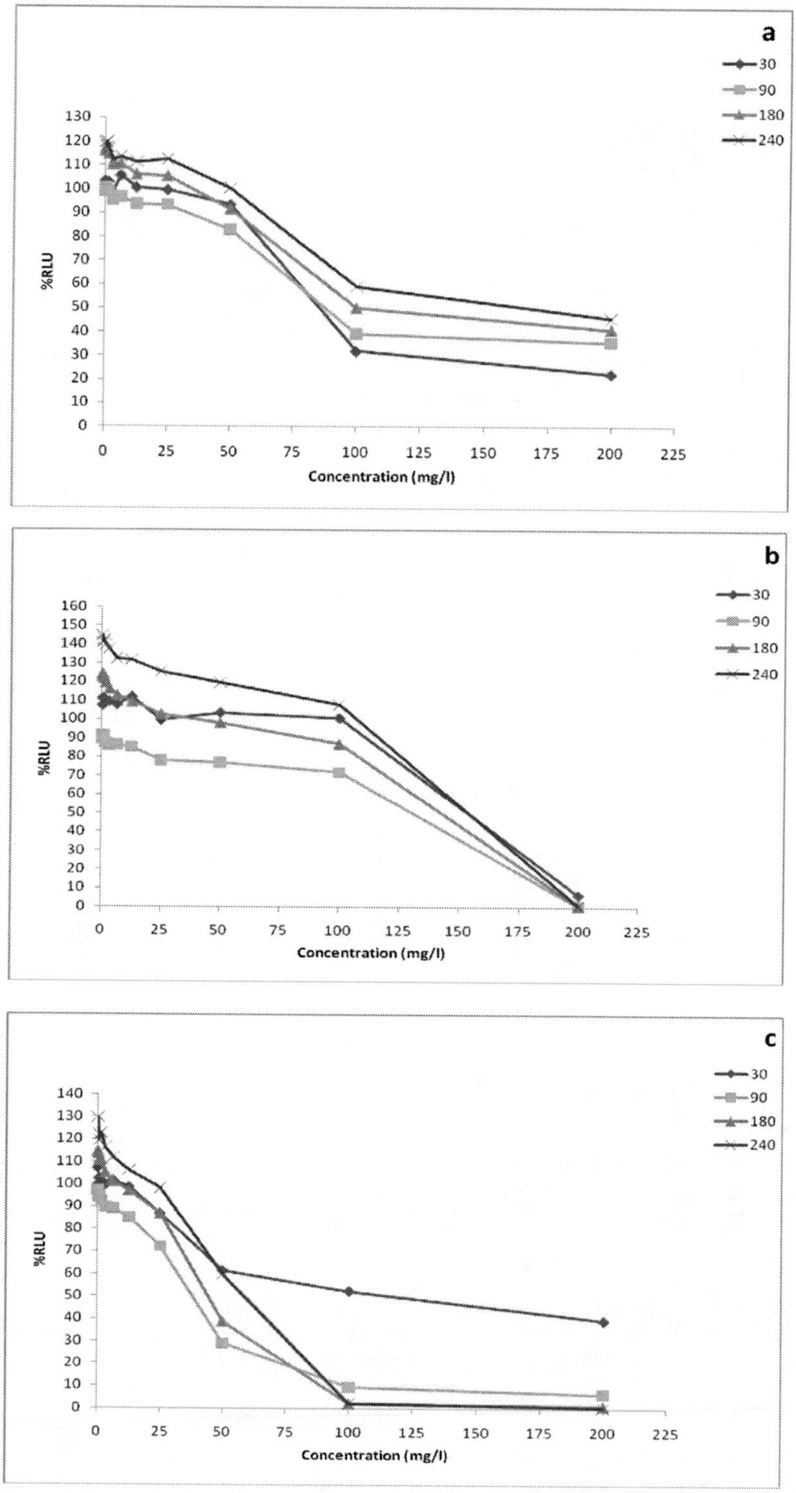

Figure 8. Light output reduction by P. putida BS566::luxCDABE when challenged with 200mg L^{-1} Ag nanoparticles (a) without stabilizer), (b) with 0.1% Citric acid and (c) with BSA after 30, 90, 80 and 240 min. Mean of three replicates with different batches. Coefficient of variation between 2 and 13% among independent assays.

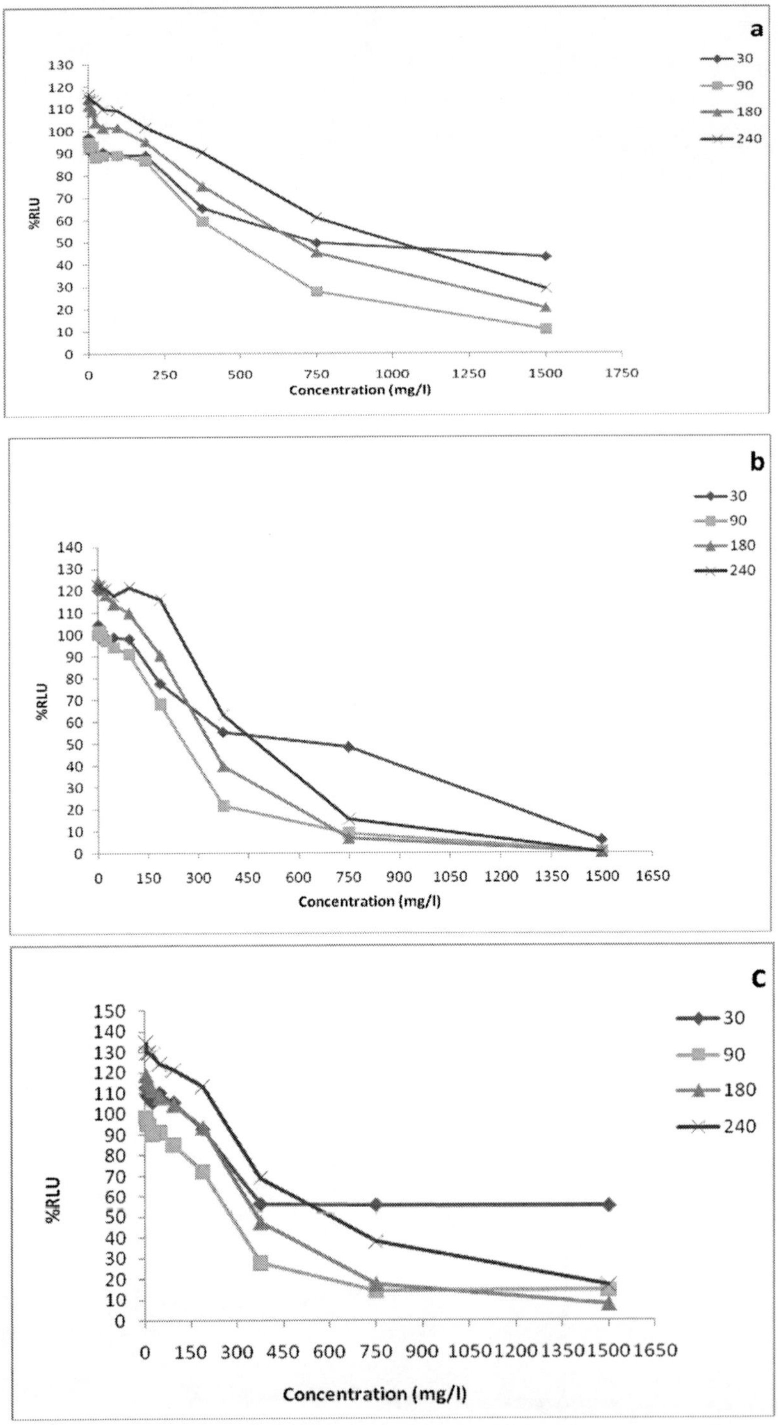

Figure 9. Light output reduction by P. putida BS566::luxCDABE when challenged with 1500mg L^{-1} Ag micro particles (a) without stabilizer), (b) with 0.1% Citric acid and (c) with BSA after 30, 90, 80 and 240 min. Mean of three replicates with different batches. Coefficient of variation between 4 and 14% among independent assays.

Silver is classified as the "soft" metal group (Blaser et al., 2008) and it complexes with many organic or inorganic materials such as chloride, sulphide, thiosulphate (Ratte, 1999). Thus, understanding the fate and transport of silver in waste water treatment plants is relevant in evaluating the impact of silver discharge in the environment and in developing a program for silver pollution control. Wastewater treatment plants are the final step to control silver discharge and our results demonstrate that the use of a bacterial biosensor as P. putida BS566::luxCDABE, native from a highly polluted environment, provides a robust, early warning system of acute toxicity which could lead to process failure. This strain is suitable for toxicity monitoring in a highly polluted industrial waste water treatment streams, including the ones with the presence of metals as silver. Silver NPs have become one of the nanomaterials most used in consumer product (Maynard and Michelson, 2006), it is considered as the most prevalent of engineered materials (Rejeski and Lekas, 2008) and is likely that nanowaste should increase and therefore enter the wastewater treatment plants. Blaser et al., (2008) pointed out that silver released to wastewater is incorporated into sewage sludge and may spread further on agricultural fields where will mainly stay in the top layer of soils (Hou et al., 2005). Landfilling of sewage sludge may allow silver to leach into subsoil and groundwater. Estimation of silver load in sewage sludge and its microorganisms growth inhibition has been predicted. Blaser et al., (2008) predicted that an expected silver concentration in sewage treatment plant range from 2 $\mu g\ L^{-1}$ to 18 $\mu g\ L^{-1}$. Shafer et al., (1998) reported a range of ~ 2 to 4 $\mu g\ L^{-1}$ of silver in sewage treatment plants treating common wastewater and a much higher load from industrial discharges (from 24 to 105 μg L-1).

The removal of silver ion by chloride free sludge is dependent on the silver-sludge loading, the solution pH and the concentration of dissolved organic matter. Studying the interactions of silver with wastewater constituents, Wang et al., (2003) showed that silver ion, under field conditions, can be removed through precipitation with chloride and adsorption by sludge particulates which increased in acidic conditions but decreased in alkaline conditions. However, the authors (Wang et al., 2003) pointed out that the formation of silver-ion-dissolved organic matter complexes, which is increased in alkaline conditions, reduces the silver ion adsorption by sludge.

Table 3. IC_{50} (mgL^{-1}) values for light emission reduction by P. putida BS566::luxCDABE after 30, 90, 180 and 240 min

Time (min)	30	90	180	240
$AgNO_3$	0.44	0.18	0.25	0.30
Ag NP	88	81	91.5	184
Ag NP –BSA	102	35	43	50
Ag NP –CA	147	126	136	149
Ag MP	715	530	765	1075
Ag MP – BSA	375	256	308	330
Ag MP- CA	700	240	300	337

Values presented are an average of at least 3 independent experiments carried out with different batches, standard deviation between 1 and 15%.

The information regarding the inhibition of microbial growth by different Ag species, especially in wastewater treatment systems, is valuable for operating planning and control. The presence and activity of microorganisms in biological wastewater treatment are vital to the process. One of the projected applications of such strains is its combined use as analytical panel for toxicant detection.

CONCLUSION

An important advantage of using this organism is that a positive response will not only indicate the presence of a toxicant but will also provide some idea as to its character.

In conclusion, our results demonstrate that the use of a bacterial biosensor as P. putida BS566::luxCDABE, native from a highly polluted environment, provides a robust, early warning system of acute toxicity which could lead to process failure. This strain is suitable for toxicity monitoring in a highly polluted industrial waste water treatment streams and it has the potential to inform on upstream process changes prior to their impacting upon the biological remediation section. Furthermore, as this reporter organism is based upon microorganisms naturally resident within the system, there remains the potential for its in situ deployment within the system with minimal effects upon their physiology.

ACKNOWLEDGMENTS

This work was part of a project funded by the Brazilian National Research and Development Council (CNPq). Also we would like to acknowledge the Environmental Research Laboratory at Edinburgh Napier University, Edinburgh, Scotland.

REFERENCES

Arnold S.M., Hickey W.J., Harris R.F. (1995). Degradation of atrazine by Fenton's reagent: Condition optimization and product quantification. *Environ. Sci. Technol.* 29, 2083-2089.

Aruoja, V., Dubourguiera, H-C., Kasemetsa, K., Kahrua, A., 2009. Toxicity of nanoparticles of CuO, ZnO and TiO2 to microalgae *Pseudokirchneriella subcapitata. Sci. Total Environ.* 407, 1461-1468.

Auffan, M., Achouak, W., Rose, J., Roncato, R-A., Chaneac, C., Waite, D.T., Maison, A., Oicik, J.C., Wiesner, M.R., Vesbottero, J-Y. (2008). Relation between the Redox State of Iron-Based Nanoparticles and Their Cytotoxicity toward *Escherichia coli. Environ. Sci. Technol. 42, 6730–6735.*

Belkin,S., Smulski, D.R., Vollmer,A.C., Van Dyk, T.K., Larossa, R.A. (1996). Oxidative Stress Detection with *Escherichia coli. Appl. Environ.Microbiol.*62, 2252–2256.

Belkin, S., Smulski D.R., Dadon S., Vollmer, A.C., Van Dyk, T.K., Larossa, R.A. (1997). Panel of stress-responsive luminous bacteria for the detection of selected classes of toxicants. *Water Res.* 31,3009-3016.

Belkin, S. (2007). Genetically engineered microorganisms for pollution monitoring. In: Soil and Water Pollution Monitoring, Protection and Remediation, NATO Science Series: IV: *Earth and Environmental Sciences*, Volume 69, 147-160.

Ben-Israel, O., Ben-Israel, H., Ulitzur,S. (1998). Identification and Quantification of Toxic Chemicals by Use of *Escherichia coli* Carrying *lux* Genes Fused to Stress Promoters. *Appl. Environ.Microbiol.* 64, 4346-4352.

Benitez F.J., Acero J.L., Real F.J. and Garcia J. (2003). Kinetics of photodegradation and ozonation of pentachlorophenol. *Chemosphere* 51, 651–662.

Blaser SA, Scheringer M, MacLeod M, Hungerbuhler K (2008). Estimation of cumulative aquatic exposure and risk due to silver: contribution of nano-functionalised plastics and textiles. *Sci. Total Environ. 390*, 396-409.

Blinova, I., Ivaska, A., Heinlaan, M., Mortimer, M., Kahru, A. (2010). Ecotoxicity of nanoparticles of CuO and ZnO in natural water. *Environ. Pollut.* 158, 41–47.

Boyd E., KIllham K., Mcharg A.A. (2001). Toxicity of mono-, di- and tri-chlorophenols to *lux* marked terrestrial bacteria, *Burkholderia* species *Rasc* c2 and *Pseudomonas fluorencens*. *Chemosphere*, 43, 157-166.

Brayner, R., Ferrari-Iliou, R., Brivois, N., Djediat, S., Benedetti, M.F., Fie′vet, F. (2006). Toxicological Impact Studies Based on *Escherichia coli* Bacteria in Ultrafine ZnO Nanoparticles Colloidal Medium. *Nanno Lett.* 866-870.

Brown, J.S., Rattray, E.A.S., Paton, G.I., Reid, G., Gaffor, I., Killham K. (1996). Comparative assessment of the toxicity of a papermil effluent by respiratory and luminescence based bacterial assay. *Chemosphere* 32, 1553-1561.

Bunce, N., Liu, L., Zhu, J.,Lane, D. (1997). Reaction of naphthalene and its derivatives with hydroxyl radicals in the gas phase. *Environ, Sci.Technol.* 31, 2252–2259.

Bystrzejewska-Piotrowska, G., Golimowski, J., Urban. P.L. (2009). Nanoparticles: Their potential toxicity, waste and environmental management. *Waste Manage.* 29, 2587–2595.

Castellano, J.J., Shafii, S.M., Ko, F., Donate, G., Wright, T.E., Mannari, R.(2007). Comparative evaluation of silver-containing antimicrobial dressings and drugs. *International Wound Journal,* 4, 114 – 122.

Chi, J., Huang, G. (2002). A multimedia fugacity river model of pentachlorophenol in south drainage canal, China. *J. Environ. Sci..Health A* 37, 113–25.

Chen, R., Pignatello, J. (1997). Role of quinone intermediates as electron shuttles in Fenton and photoassisted Fenton oxidation of aromatic compounds. *Environ. Sci.Technol.* 31, 2399–2406.

Choi, O., Deng, K.K., Kim, N-J., Ross Jr,, L, Surampalli, R.Y., Hu, Z. (2008). The inhibitory effects of silver nanoparticles, silver ions, and silver chloride colloids on microbial growth. *Water Res*. 42, 3066-3074.

Choi, S.H., Gu, M.B. (2003). Toxicity biomonitoring of degradation byproducts using freeze-dried recombinant bioluminescent bacteria. *Chimica Acta* 481, 229–238.

Chu, C.L., Lin,P.H., Dong, Y.S., Guo, D.Y. (2002). Influences of citric acid as a chelating reagent on the characteristics of nanophase hydroxyapatite powders fabricated by a sol-gel method. *J. Mat. Sci. Lett.* 21, 1793-1795.

Copley, S.D. (2000). Evolution of a metabolic pathway for degradation of a toxic xenobiotic: the patchwork approach. *Trends Biochem.Sci.*25, 261-265.

Cronin, M.T.D., Schultz, T.W.(1998). Structure–Toxicity Relationships for Three Mechanisms of Action of Toxicity to *Vibrio fischeri*. (1998). *Ecotoxicol. Environ. Saf.* 39, 65-69.

Damianovic, M.H.R.Z., Moraes, E.M., Zaiat, M., Foresti E. (2009). Pentachlorophenol (PCP) dechlorination in horizontal-flow anaerobic immobilized biomass (HAIB) reactors. *Bioresource Technol.*100, 4361–4367.

Dennison, M.J., Turner, A.P.F. (1995). Biosensors for environmental monitoring. *Biotechnol. Adv.* 13, 1-12.

Eker, S., Kargi, F. (2007). Performance of a hybrid-loop bioreactor system in biological treatment of 2,4,6-trichlorophenol containing synthetic wastewater: effects of hydraulic residence time. *J. Hazard. Mater.* 144, 86–92.

Escher, B.I., Snozzi, M., Schwarzenbach, R.P. (1996). Uptake, speciation and uncoupling activity of substituted phenols in energy transducing membranes. *Environ. Sci. Technol.* 30, 3071-3079.

Fallmann, H., Krutzler, R., Bauer, S., Blanco, M.J. (1999). Applicability of the Photo-Fenton method for treating water containing pesticides. *Catal. Today* 54, 309-319.

Foucaud, L., Wilson, M.R., Brown, D.M.,Stone, V. (2007). Measurements of reactive species production by nanoparticles prepared in biologically relevant media. *Toxicol. Lett.* 174, 1-9.

Fukushima, M., Kawasaki, M., Sawada, A., Ichikawa, H., Morimoto, K., Tatsumi, K., Tanaka, S. (2002). Facilitation of pentachlorophenol degradation by the addition of ascorbic acid to aqueous mixtures of tetrakis(sulfonatophenyl) porphyrin and iron(II) *J. Mol. Catal A- Chem* 187, 201–213.

Gomez, M., Murcia,M.D., Gomez, E., Gomez, J.L., Dams, R., Christofi, N. (2010). Enhancement of 4-Chlorophenol Photodegradation with KrCl Excimer UV Lamp by Adding Hydrogen Peroxide. *Separ. Sci. Technol.* 45, 1603–1609.

Gorska, P., Zaleska, A., Hupka, J. (2009). Photodegradation of phenol by UV/TiO2 and Vis/N,C-TiO2 processes: Comparative mechanistic and kinetic studies. *Sep. Purif. Technol.* 68, 90–96.

Gu, M.B., Choi, S.H. (2001). Monitoring and classification of toxicity using recombinant bioluminescent bacteria. *Water Sci. Technol.* 43, 147–154.

Hirvonen, A., Trapido, M., Hentunen, J., Tarhanen, J. (2000). Formation of hydroxylated and dimeric intermediates during oxidation of chlorinated phenols in aqueous solutions. *Chemosphere* 41, 1211–1218.

Heinlaan, M., Ivask, A., Blinova, I., Dubourguier, H-C., Kahru, A. (2008). Toxicity of nanosized and bulk ZnO, CuO and TiO2 to bacteria Vibrio fischeri and crustaceans Daphnia magna and Thamnocephalus platyurus. *Chemosphere,* 71, 1308-1316.

Hollender, J., Hopp, J., Dott, W. (1997). Degradation of 4-Chlorophenol via the *meta* Cleavage Pathway by *Comamonas testosteroni* JH5. *Appl. Environ. Microbiol.* 63, 4567–4572.

Hong A.P.K., Zeng Y. (2002). Degradation of pentachlorophenol by ozonation and biodegradability of intermediates. *Water Res.* 36, 4243–4254.

Hou, H., Takamatsu, T., Koshikawa, M.K., Hosomi, M. (2005). Migration of silver, indium, tin, antimony and bismuth and variations in their chemical fractions on addition to uncontaminated soils. *Soil Sci.* 170, 624-639.

Jiang, W., Mashayekhi, H., Xing, B. (2009). Bacterial toxicity comparison between nano- and micro-scaled oxide particles. *Environ. Poll.* 157,1619–1625.

Kang, N., Lee, D.S., Yoon, J. (2002). Kinetic modelling of Fenton oxidation of phenol and monochlorophenols. *Chemosphere,* 47, 915–924.

Keith, L.H., Telliard, W.A. (1979). Priority pollutants: a prospective view. *Environ. Sci. Technol.* 13,416–424.

Kim, J., Kuk, E., Yu, K., Kim, J., Park, S., Lee, H., Kim, S., Park, Y., Park, C., Wang, C. (2007). Antimicrobial effects of silver nanoparticles. *Nanomedicine: Nanotechnology, Biology and Medicine,* 3, 95-101.

Landsdown, A.B.C.(2002). Silver I: its antibacterial properties and mechanism of action. *J. Wound Care*, 11:125-138.

Leppard, G.G., Mavrocordatos, D., Perret, D. (2003).Electron-optical characterization of nano- and micro-particles in raw and treated waters: an overview. In: Boller M, editor. Proceedings of nano and microparticles in water and wastewater treatment, 50 (12). *Water Sci Technol,* 1–8.

Litchfield, C.D., Rao, M. (1998). Pentachlorophenol biodegradation:laboratory and field studies. In: *Biological treatment of hazardous wastes.* (L.J. DeFilippi, Ed). Wiley, New York, pp. 271–283.

Luo, T., Ai Z., Zhang, L. (2008). Fe@Fe2O3 core-shell nanowires as iron reagent 4 Sono-Fenton degradation of pentachlorophenol and the mechanism analysis. *Journal of Physics and Chemistry* 112, 8675–8681.

Madsen, T., Aamand, J. (1990). Effects of sulforoxy anions on degradation of pentachlorophenol by a methanogenic enrichment culture. *Appl. Environ. Microbiol.* 57, 2453–2458.

Maynard, A.D., Michelson, E. (2006). *The Nanotechnology Consumer Product Inventory* (http://nanotechnproject.org/44).

McAllister, K.A., Lee, H., Trevors, J.T. (1996). *Microbial degradation of pentachlorophenol. Biodegradation.* 7, 1–40.

Miller, R.M., Singer, G.M., Rosen, J.D., Bartha, R. (1988). Sequential degradation of chlorophenols by photolytic and microbial treatment. *Environ. Sci. Technol.* 22, 1215 - 1219.

Mills, G., Hoffmann, M.R. (1993). Photocatalytic degradation of pentachlorophenol on TiO2 particles: Identification of intermediates and mechanism of reaction. *Environ. Sci.Technol.* 27, 1681-1689.

Mortimer, M., Kasemets, K., Kurvet, I., Heinlaan, M., Kahru, A. (2008). Kinetic Vibrio fischeri bioluminescence inhibition assay for study of toxic effects of nanoparticles and colored/turbid samples. *Toxicol. in Vitro*, 22, 1412-1417.

Pal, S., Tak, Y.K., Song, J.M. (2007). Does the antibacterial activity of silver nanoparticles depend upon the shape of the nanoparticle? A study of the Gram-negative bacterium *Escherichia coli. Appl. Environ. Microbiol.* 73, 1712–1720.

Paton, G.I., Campbell, C.D., Glover, L.A., Killham, K. (1995). Assessment of bioavailability of heavy metals using lux modified constructs of *Pseudomonas fluorescens. Lett. Appl. Microbiol.* 20, 52–56.

Paton, G.I., Palmer, G., Burton, M., Rattray, E.A., McGrath, S.P., Killham K. (1997). Development of an acute and chronic ecotoxicity assay using *lux*-marked *Rhizobium leguminosarum* biovar *trifoli. Lett.Appl.Microbiol.* 24, 296-300.

Paulus, W. (1993). *Microbiocides for the protection of materials*.London, Chapman & Hall, London, United Kingdom, 526pp.

Pera-Titus, M., Garcia-Molina, V., Ban′ os, M., Gimenez, J., Esplugas, S. (2004). Degradation of chlorophenols by means of advanced oxidation processes: a general review. *Appl.Catal B- Environ.* 47, 219–256.

Ratte, H.T. (1999). Bioaccumulation and toxicity of silver compounds: a review. *Environ. Toxicol. Chem.* 18, 89-108.

Rejeski, D., Lekas, D. (2008). Nanotechnology field observations: scouting the new industrial waste. *J. Cleaner Prod.* 16, 1014-1017.

Shafer, M.M., Overdier, J.T., Armstong, D.H. (1998). Removal portioning and fate of silver and other metals in wastewater treatment plants and effluent-receiving streams. Environ. *Toxicol. Chem.* 17(4), 630-641.

Siejak, P., Frackowiak, D. (2007). Interactions between colloidal silver and photosynthetic pigments located in cyanobacteria fragments and in solution. *J. Photochem.Photobio B.* 88, 126-130.

Sinha, R., Karan, R., Sinha, A., Khare, S.K. (in press). Interaction and nanotoxic effect of ZnO and Ag nanoparticles on mesophilic and halophilic bacterial cells. *Bioresour. Technol.* (2010), doi:10.1016/j.biortech.2010.07.117.

Slabbert, J.L. (1986). Improved bacterial growth test for rapid water toxicity screening. *Bull. Environ. Contam. Toxicol.* 37, 565–569.

Sondi, I., Salopek-Sondi,B. (2004). Silver nanoparticles as antimicrobial agent: a case study on *E. coli* as a model for Gram-negative bacteria. *J.Colloid. Interf. Sci.* 275, 177-182.

Stefan, M.I., Bolton, J.R. (1998). Mechanism of the degradation of 1,4-dioxane in dilute aqueous solution using the UV/ hydrogen peroxide process. *Environ. Sci. Technol.* 32, 1588-1595.

Sundstrom, D.W., Weir, B.A., Klei, H.E. (1989). Destruction of aromatic pollutants by UV light catalyzed oxidation with hydrogen peroxide. *Environ. Prog.* 8, 6-11.

Wang, J., Huan, C.P., Pirestan, D. (2003). Interactions of silver with wastewater constituents. *Water Res.* 37, 4444-4452.

Weavers, L., Malsmatdt, N., Hoffman, M. (2000). Kinetics and mechanism of pentachlorophenol by sonication, ozonation, and sonolytics ozonation. *Environ. Sci. Technol.* 34, 1280–1285.

Westerhoff, P., Zhang, Y., Crittenden, J., Chen, Y.(2008). Properties of commercial nanoparticles that affect their removal during water treatment. In: Grassian VH, editor. Nanoscience and Nanotechnology*: Environmental and Health Impacts.* NJ: John Wiley and Sons, 71–90.

Whiteley, A.S., Wiles, S., Lilley, A.K., Philp, J., Bailey, M.J. (2001). Ecological and physiological analyses of Pseudomonad species within a phenol remediation system. *J. Microbiol. Meth.* 44, 79– 88.

Wiles, S., Whiteley, A.S., Philp, J.C., Bailey, M.J. (2003). Development of bespoke bioluminescent reporters with the potential for in situ deployment within a phenolic-remediating wastewater treatment system. *J. Microbiol. Meth.* 55, 667– 677.

Winson, M., Swift, S., Hill, P.J., Sims, C.M., Griesmayr, G., Bycroft, B.W., Williams, P., Gordon, S.A.B., Stewart, G.S.A.B. (1998). Engineering the luxCDABE genes from *Photorhabdus luminescens* to provide a bioluminescent reporter for constitutive and promoter probe plasmids and mini-Tn5 constructs. *FEMS Microbiol. Lett.* 163,193-202.

Wu, W.M., Hickey, R.F., Bhatnagar, M.K., Zeikus, J.C. (1989). Fatty acid degradation as a toll to monitor anaerobic sludge activity and toxicity. In: *44th Purdue University Industrial Waste Conference Proceedings*, pp. 225–233.

Zeng, Y., Wackett, L. (2008). Pentachlorophenol Family Pathway Map. http://umbbd.ethz.ch/pcp/pcp_map.html. 16/06/2010.

Zhao, G., Stevens, E. (1998). Multiple parameters for the comprehensive evaluation of the susceptibility of *Escherichia coli* to the silver ion. *BioMetals*, 11, 27-32.

INDEX

B

C

D

F

G

H

I

J

K

L

M

N

O

Q

R

S

T

U

V

W

X

Y

Z